Comprehensive Manuals of Surgical Specialties

Richard H. Egdahl, editor

Manual of Vascular Surgery, Volume I
Edwin J. Wylie/Ronald J. Stoney/William K. Ehrenfeld

Errata

Some errors regrettably occur in this volume, and Springer-Verlag apologizes for any inconvenience these may cause. The following list describes how the text *should* read, with the precise change, from the existing text, printed in italics.

page 12, **Fig. 2.3,a,b.** Should read:

"Clamping an atherosclerotic artery. **a** *incorrect* angle; **b** *correct* angle."

page 31, **Fig. 2.29b.** Should read:

"**b** Demonstration of two potential endarterectomy planes by passage of a clamp behind a central core of atheroma. The plane at the *bottom* is the preferred one in most situations. The plane at the *top* has been developed within the atheromatous intima."

page 72, third paragraph, beginning in line 2: Should read:

"The cul-de-sac in the artery is filled with blood to displace any air bubbles *by* releasing the clamp on the shunt."

page 78, **Fig. 3.46b** is printed upside down.

page 80, **Fig. 3.48,** beginning in line 2: Should read:

"Thrombosis occurred as the result of progression to occlusion of an atheroma at the common carotid bifurcation (*left*)."

Edwin J. Wylie   Ronald J. Stoney   William K. Ehrenfeld

Manual of Vascular Surgery

Volume I

Includes 557 illustrations,
471 in full color

Illustrated by Ted Bloodhart

Springer-Verlag
New York   Heidelberg   Berlin

SERIES EDITOR

Richard H. Egdahl, M.D., Ph.D., Professor of Surgery, Boston University Medical Center, Boston, Massachusetts 02118

AUTHORS

Edwin J. Wylie, M.D., Professor of Surgery, Chief, Vascular Surgery Service, School of Medicine, University of California, San Francisco, California 94143

Ronald J. Stoney, M.D., Professor of Surgery, Vascular Surgery Service, School of Medicine, University of California, San Francisco, California 94143

William K. Ehrenfeld, M.D., Associate Professor of Surgery, Vascular Surgery Service, School of Medicine, University of California, San Francisco, California 94143

MEDICAL ILLUSTRATOR

Ted Bloodhart, 1136 West Sixth Street, Los Angeles, California 90017

Library of Congress Cataloging in Publication Data

Wylie, Edwin J.   1918–
   Manual of vascular surgery (v. I).
   (Comprehensive manuals of surgical specialties)
   Includes index.
   1. Blood-vessels—Surgery.   I. Stoney, Ronald J., joint author.   II. Ehrenfeld, William K., 1934—joint author.   III. Title. [DNLM: 1. Vascular surgery —Handbooks. WG170 W983n]
RD598.5.W93   617'.414   79-18226

Printed in the United States of America.

9 8 7 6 5 4 3 2 1

ISBN 0-387-90408-5   Springer-Verlag   New York   Heidelberg   Berlin
ISBN 3-540-90408-5   Springer-Verlag   Berlin   Heidelberg   New York

To

Maile Ota, R.N.

in appreciation of her twenty years of loyal support to the
Vascular Surgery Service, and in recognition of her effective
teaching of both resident surgeons and surgical nurses.

Editor's Note

Comprehensive Manuals of Surgical Specialties is a series of surgical manuals designed to present current operative techniques and to explore various aspects of diagnosis and treatment. The series features a unique format with emphasis on large, detailed, full-color illustrations, schematic charts, and photographs to demonstrate integral steps in surgical procedures.

Each manual focuses on a specific region or topic and describes surgical anatomy, physiology, pathology, diagnosis, and operative treatment. Operative techniques and stratagems for dealing with surgically correctable disorders are described in detail. Illustrations are primarily depicted from the surgeon's viewpoint to enhance clarity and comprehension.

Other volumes in preparation:

Manual of Cardiac Surgery
Manual of Liver Surgery
Manual of Soft Tissue Tumor Surgery
Manual of Upper Gastrointestinal Surgery
Manual of Ambulatory Surgery
Manual of Trauma Surgery

Richard H. Egdahl

vii

Preface

Of all the developing fields of surgery, few have had the impact of vascular surgery in affecting so large a segment of the population with its potential for relief of disability or the prolongation of life. As would be anticipated, the interest of surgeons in this evolving specialty has been largely focused upon the selection of the most appropriate operations and the development of modifications or new procedures to overcome the limitations of previous ones.

The literature contains numerous conflicting claims on the relative merits of various procedures. Those approaching this field for the first time may understandably be confused. Yet, if one were to approach any single vascular surgeon at any given time, he would, upon request, receive a firm and precise listing of preferred procedures.

The procedures described in this two-volume publication are those which we currently favor. Their selection is the result of continuing analysis of our own experience of the last 25 years. All patients have been available for prolonged follow-up evaluation. Late failures often identified techniques that lessened the durability of initially satisfactory operations and stimulated the development of modifications or trials with alternate operations. Particular attention is directed here to the manner in which knowledge of the natural history of disease influences the choice of operation.

Volume I presents an initial chapter on arteriography as it relates to the vascular surgeon. The second chapter deals with the basic principles of vascular reconstructive techniques. Both chapters present material applicable to subsequent portions of both volumes dealing with specific clinical entities. The remaining chapters deal with arterial reconstructive techniques as they relate to atherosclerotic lesions of the major arteries (exclusive of the femoropopliteal segments).

The common denominators in many of the clinical aspects as well as technical requirements of arterial reconstruction as they apply to atherosclerosis in every location suggested a pathologic rather than a regional grouping of subject matter. Surgical considerations in atherosclerosis of the arteries in the lower extremities as well as other conditions and diseases in all regions will be presented in the Volume II of this work.

We have attempted to combine a descriptive manual with an illustrative atlas. Pertinent clinical considerations that lead to decisions for or against operation and the selection of the most appropriate operation are discussed. Particular emphasis is placed upon the preoperative and intraoperative recognition of pathologic variations which may require modification of a planned procedure or the selection of an alternate one. Insofar as is possible, these variations are illustrated by appropriate arteriograms and photographs of surgical specimens.

The exposition of each operation uses sequential drawings and is designed to illustrate successive steps in the technical maneuvers. We are particularly indebted to Mr. Ted Bloodhart for his skill and imagination in the selection of illustrative techniques and for the clarity of the drawings.

Contents

Arteriography

Arteriography is necessary for preoperative diagnosis and operative planning in most patients for whom arterial reconstructive surgery may become necessary. The safety of most currently employed techniques has reached the level where arteriography is often the first study performed after the original clinical evaluation. Although a variety of "noninvasive" techniques are currently under study, none has supplanted arteriography for precision of diagnosis. This chapter categorizes the various arteriographic techniques in terms of their usefulness to the surgeon, describes those situations where one method may be safer and more accurate than another, and calls attention to specific precautions.

Cerebrovascular Disease

Indications for cerebral arteriography in patients under study for possible cerebrovascular disease are listed in **Tables 1.1 and 1.2.** The preferable method is the Seldinger technique with introduction of the catheter in one common femoral artery. Hemorrhage from the puncture site after removal of the catheter can be effectively controlled by manual compression for 10–15 min on the groin supplemented with sandbag compression for 2–3 hours. The patient is cautioned to remain supine for the next 12 hours. We have never encountered a bleeding problem from the puncture site after this time.

If proximal passage of the catheter is impeded at the iliac level, the catheter should be promptly withdrawn and reinserted into the opposite femoral artery. If difficulty is again encountered, the femoral approach should be abandoned. Further attempts invite an intramural dissection and the potential for arterial occlusion. In patients who have symptoms and findings of substantial iliofemoral atherosclerosis for which abdominal aortography will also be required, we prefer to precede the cerebrovascular study with a translumbar aortogram to aid in the selection of the most appropriate femoral artery for safe introduction of a catheter or to determine whether the femoral route should be abandoned in favor of another approach.

TABLE 1.1.   Indications and Contraindications for Arteriography in Suspected Cerebrovascular Occlusive Disease

Indicated

   A.   If needed for differential diagnosis

      Aneurysm
      Angioma
      Tumor
      Subdural hematoma
      Focal epileptic attacks
      Subarachnoid hemorrhage

   B.   If operation would be advisable if a surgically accessible arterial lesion were demonstrated

Contraindicated

Recent cerebral infarction (30 days)

The second choice of a site for insertion of the catheter is the axillary artery. This route is less desirable than the femoral because of greater difficulty in positioning the catheter for selective carotid injection. When the catheter is inserted through the axilla, one may often have to settle for a simple injection of the aortic arch. The axillary artery is also more vulnerable to a lengthy tear, and manual compression is more difficult to apply effectively. An occasional patient may develop problems secondary to injury to the brachial plexus.

Injection of the brachial artery is not advised because of the greater risk of local thrombosis when the catheter is removed. Injection of the subclavian artery, a technique formerly used, introduces the unnecessary risk of pneumothorax. Percutaneous needle injection of the common carotid arteries, one of the original techniques for visualization of the carotid territory, has been largely discarded for patients with suspected cerebrovascular disease because of the risk of intramural dissection or disruption of an atheromatous plaque in a low-lying bifurcation. In addition, extramural hemorrhage following removal of the needle often dissects for a lengthy distance within the carotid sheath. The resulting soft-tissue reaction creates problems for the surgeon in identifying and preserving vital structures, e.g., the vagus or hypoglossal nerves, if a subsequent carotid operation is required.

The extent of visualization of the extra- and intracranial arteries is determined by diagnostic needs. Neurotoxicity of the contrast solutions currently in use, although substantially less than those formerly used, is still a consideration and is related in part to the total volume used and its concentration. The early concept that visualization of the aortic arch branches, the four cervical arteries supplying the brain and their intracranial tributaries, was necessary for an adequate evaluation of patients with suspected occlusive cerebrovascular disease has been replaced by more selective studies based upon the required therapy if a suspected lesion is demonstrated. Thus, for patients with symptoms or findings in the carotid territory alone, selective carotid injections of the intracranial branches is usually adequate. A separate arch injection in two projections is required (1) in patients with findings suggesting subclavian, innominate, or proximal vertebral disease *only if the demonstration of lesions at this level would indicate the need for operation* or (2) when the radiologist encounters difficulty in catheterizing the carotid arteries. An arch study alone for suspected carotid disease is often difficult to interpret because of overlapping arteries both in the neck and intracranially.

TABLE 1.2.   Indications for Arteriography when Diagnosis of Cerebrovascular Occlusive Disease Is Probable

  I.   Symptoms of *Transient Cerebral Ischemia*

Carotid territory	Lateralizing motor or sensory deficits
	Expressive dysphasia
	Monocular visual loss

Vertebro-basilar territory	Vertigo
	Ataxia
	Diplopia
	Slurred speech
	Drop attacks
	Bilateral visual impairment

 II.   *Persistent or Recurrent Symptoms of Decreased Cerebral Perfusion* (postural dizziness, blurred vision)

After excluding or correcting
  a.   Anemia
  b.   Postural hypotension
  c.   Inadequate cardiac output

and physical findings suggest
  a.   Stenosis at carotid bifurcation
  b.   Stenosis or occlusion of:
      (1)   Common carotid artery
      *(2)   Subclavian or innominate arteries

III.   *Asymptomatic Patients Whose Vascular Findings Indicate Neurologic Jeopardy*
  a.   Unilateral carotid bruit when major thoracic or abdominal surgery is anticipated
  b.   Bilateral carotid bifurcation bruits
  c.   Absent common carotid pulse

* Indication for study related to degree of disability.

When embolization from a cervical carotid lesion is suspected, two or even three projections are usually necessary to demonstrate the contour of the arterial lumen adequately. If right hemispheric embolization is suspected and the carotid studies are normal, an arch injection is required to demonstrate the innominate artery, in which ulcerating lesions may also occur. An arch injection in two projections is adequate to demonstrate vertebral lesions. Selective injection of the vertebral arteries carries a prohibitive risk. The two most disastrous complications in our experience have been acute vertebral occlusion secondary to an intramural injection and cortical blindness from perfusing the posterior circulation with essentially undiluted contrast solution. Intramural injection may also occasionally occur with selective carotid injection, but ordinarily is a benign event.

Many patients will have a history of adverse reactions from previous injection of contrast solution. In this situation we customarily initiate steroid therapy the day before the study and give an oral dose of Benadryl (50 mg) before the study is begun. Although we have an anesthetist on standby for intubation and ventilatory support, his services have never been required.

Visceral Artery Disease, Renovascular Hypertension, Portal Hypertension

Catheter arteriography is the preferred technique in most patients with symptoms suggesting visceral artery disease or renovascular hypertension. For patients with suspected celiac or superior mesenteric artery disease,

3

midstream aortic injections are made in the AP and lateral projections: the first to show the comparative rate of distal opacification and the collateral vessels; the second, to demonstrate the arteries at their origin.

For patients with suspected renovascular hypertension caused by atherosclerotic orifice lesions, multiple midstream aortic injections are usually required to demonstrate the renal arteries accurately. The renal artery orifices vary in location on the circumference of the aorta from a lateral to a postero-lateral position. Varying degrees of rotation of the patient are usually necessary to visualize the artery orifices in profile. Selective catheterization should be reserved for patients in whom the midstream injection demonstrates fibromuscular dysplasia. Arterial elongation, tortuosity, and even coiling are characteristics of this disease. Views in varying projections taken in full inspiration to depress the kidney and straighten the artery are needed to define clearly the extent of disease. Accurate anatomic definition is critically important not only for diagnosis but also to allow the surgeon to select the most appropriate operative technique. Lesions beyond the bifurcation for which *ex vivo* techniques are frequently necessary may escape detection without these more precise arteriographic techniques.

For patients with portal hypertension the preoperative determination of portal vein patency or the postoperative assessment of shunt patency (regardless of the type of the decompression operation), selective injection of the celiac artery is a particularly useful technique. The late films in the angiographic series delineate the venous pathways.

Aortoiliac or Femoropopliteal Disease

Translumbar aortography to demonstrate obstructive lesions in the infrarenal aorta, the iliac arteries, and the femoral-popliteal segments has, in our experience, been the most acceptable arteriographic technique. Atherosclerosis in these areas is usually accompanied by some degree of intimal disease in the common femoral arteries. In this situation, catheter injection of the common femoral artery creates the potential for local thrombosis requiring immediate surgical correction. Cephalad passage of the catheter adds the risk of intimal disruption at a higher level. Although these complications are rare, their occasional occurences are predictable. In addition, the inevitable periarterial hematoma in the groin complicates the technical performance of an aortofemoral graft or endarterectomy, should one of these operations become necessary. Catheter injection of a fabric graft in the groin for patients who have developed recurrent symptoms after a previous aortofemoral graft operation is particularly hazardous. The interior of such a graft, particularly when it is larger than the outflow tract, is lined by a layer of thin, loosely attached thrombus that is vulnerable to disruption or thrombosis, which the traumatic insertion of a catheter would cause.

Translumbar aortography avoids all these problems. In more than 9000 cases by this method in our clinic, there have been only three genuine complications. Two occurred as a result of hemorrhage from the wall of an infrarenal false aneurysm of the aorta, and one was a result of an intramural injection occluding a severely diseased distal aorta, for which immediate operation was required. When an adequate volume of contrast solution has been injected and with proper timing of film exposures, visualization of the arterial tree to at least the level of the midcalf can be obtained.

For patients with an abdominal aortic aneurysm or occlusion of the aorta to the level of the renal arteries, translumbar aortography is less effective in demonstrating the distal arterial tree. In the case of the former, the combination of low flow velocity and dilution of contrast solution in the dilated aorta and iliac segments lessens opacification in the distal arteries to a degree that adequate visualization of the more distal vessels is rarely obtained. Since it is so rare that the clinical problem requires distal arteriography, this drawback is more theoretical than real. In almost every instance of combined aneurysmal and occlusive disease, selection of the most appropriate grafting technique can be made at the time of operation.

In patients with subrenal aortic occlusion, translumbar aortography frequently fails to provide adequate visualization of the distal arterial tree. A large portion of the collateral supply to the legs supplied by the superior mesenteric artery (by way of the meandering mesenteric–inferior mesenteric–obturator connections) is so diluted by the distal inflow of blood from the circumflex iliac and inferior epigastric arteries that distal opacification may be inadequate when contrast solution has been introduced into the proximal abdominal aorta. Fortunately this does not create a clinical problem in patient management. If the distal extent of occlusion is beyond the common femoral arteries, viability of the leg will have been lost beyond retrieval by revascularization. If the leg is viable when aortography demonstrates subrenal aortic occlusion, either the common femoral or the profunda femoris artery assuredly is patent and available for a distal graft anastomosis.

Although translumbar aortography can be performed with local anesthesia, severe pain usually occurs at the time of injection. This can be avoided by the use of an epidural anesthetic, which has been our technique of choice. Blood pressure should be maintained at the patient's customary level. A lowered pressure will reduce aortic blood flow velocity and impair visualization of the distal vessels.

Technique

With the patient in the prone position the needle is introduced in the costovertebral angle. If the needle is angled toward the opposite axilla it will penetrate the aorta at the level of the diaphragm. If the angle is in the direction of the opposite iliac crest, penetration is just proximal to the bifurcation. An angle midway between these extremes will usually position the needle in the aorta immediately distal to the renal arteries, which, except for patients with aortic aneurysms or aortic occlusion at the level of the renal arteries, is the most suitable site for injection. If clinical findings suggest aortic occlusion, a dry tap at this site indicates occlusion to the renal artery level and the need for reinsertion of the needle at a higher level.

A 17-gauge dos Santos needle, which has side holes proximal to the occluded tip, is used (**Fig. 1.1,** stylet partially withdrawn). A needle with an open beveled tip will occasionally produce an intramural dissection when a portion of the opening is within the aortic wall. Forceful injection through an open-end needle will occasionally cause the needle to withdraw from its intraluminal position.

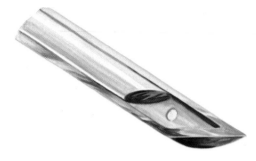

Fig. 1.1. Tip of dos Santos needle with stylet partially withdrawn.

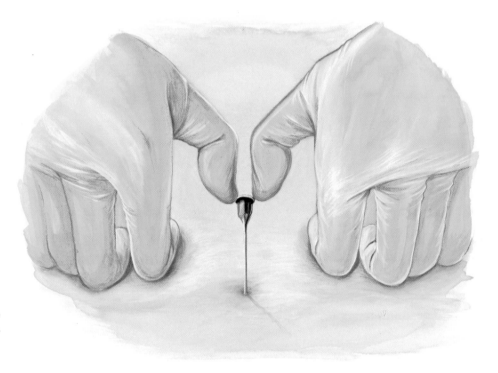

Fig. 1.2. Insertion of translumbar needle; stylet withdrawn on approach to aorta.

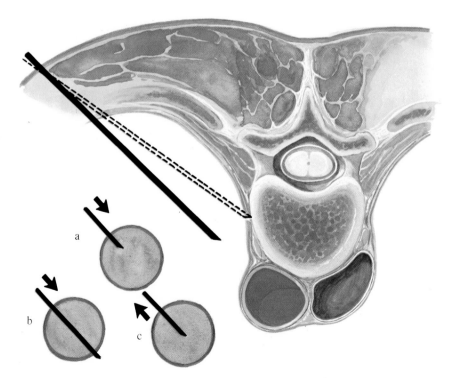

Fig. 1.3. Steps in insertion of translumbar needle.

6

The needle is inserted at an angle that directs it to the body of the lumbar vertebrae. For an infrarenal injection this angle is 60° from the vertical. For suprarenal injections the angle is 70°–75° from the vertical. The needle is then partially withdrawn and the angle lessened with each reinsertion until the needle barely clears the bone. The stylet is withdrawn and the needle is carefully advanced with the operator's knuckles against the patient's back to maintain control (**Fig. 1.2**). **Fig. 1.3** shows the introductory maneuvers. When the side holes are within the aortic lumen, a vigorous jet of blood issues from the hub of the needle (a). The needle is then advanced until bleeding ceases (b). It is then withdrawn one-half the distance of the advance to make certain that the side holes are in the center of the lumen (c). The needle is then connected to the plastic tubing leading to a pressure injector. The appearance of blood within the tubing after momentary tripping of the "load" button makes certain the needle's position has not been changed. Sixty cubic centimeters of contrast solution (Renografin-76) is injected during a 3-sec interval. Five film exposures are made at 3-sec intervals. If severe ischemia of the legs is present, exposure of the final film should be delayed for a few seconds to allow time for the contrast solution to reach the terminal popliteal branches. If the timing has been incorrect, a second injection can be made without risk to the patient.

Basic Techniques in Arterial Reconstruction

2

A little neglect may breed mischief: For want of a
nail the shoe was lost; for want of a shoe the horse
was lost; and for want of a horse the rider was lost.

A maxim from George Herbert prefixed to
Poor Richard's Almanac, Benjamin Franklin, 1757

There are few surgical disciplines to which the above adage applies as
well as to vascular surgery. Imperfect exposure, careless handling of diseased vessels, neglect in clot prevention, and improper suture techniques
are but a few of the multitude of errors that lead to failure that so often
means loss of an extremity, paralysis, or death. This chapter illustrates and
describes a variety of basic principles in vascular reconstructive surgery
that apply to the operations described in subsequent chapters.

Exposure

The development of adequate exposure is usually the most time-consuming and often the most demanding portion of the operation. The afferent
and efferent vessels on both sides of the diseased arterial segments must be
easily available for safe clamp control without impinging upon the segment
to be resected and/or repaired. Hence the full-length sternotomy incision
for innominate endarterectomy or bypass, the full-length abdominal incision for operation on lesions at the aortic bifurcation, the thoracoretroperitoneal approach for suprarenal aortic disease, and even the partial transection of the inguinal ligament for aortofemoral grafting operations. The
selection of the proper approach should also take into account the possibility that an operation more extensive than the one originally proposed may
become necessary. A lower-quadrant extraperitoneal approach for apparent unilateral iliac artery disease may often be disastrous when the surgeon finds it necessary to control or repair the aorta or the contralateral
common iliac artery.

Arterial or Venous Mobilization

Use of slings encircling the arteries or veins is a necessary vascular retraction technique. Use of fabric slings (e.g., hernia or umbilical tapes) is discouraged as they often become ensnarled in the adventitia as they are passed behind the vessel, so they twist the vessel as they are passed around it (**Fig. 2.1a and b**). Because the fabric narrows at its point of contact with the artery when traction is applied, the friable intima in a patient with atherosclerosis may be fractured at this point and becomes a nidus for thrombosis or the origin of a postoperative dissection (**Fig. 2.1c and d**).

Soft rubber tubing, cut to a point and moistened, slides easily around the vessel and holds its shape when subjected to the minor degree of traction required, thereby avoiding both difficulties described above (**Fig. 2.2a and b**). For large and medium-sized arteries, latex tubing with an external diameter of $^3/_{16}$ in. is used.[1] Smaller rubber or plastic tubing strips are now commercially available for use on smaller arteries such as the branches of the profunda femoris or the subclavian arteries. The use of two slings permits elevation of an arterial segment with minimal distortion of the artery as the loose periarterial fibrous tissue is dissected away from the artery (**Fig. 2.2c**).

Arterial Occlusion

The temporary interruption of blood flow is necessary in most vascular reconstructive operations and may be accomplished by tourniquets, vascular clamps, or intra-arterial balloon catheters. In patients with atherosclerosis, particular care is required to prevent the creation of a new lesion by the occlusion technique. Although the atherosclerotic lesion that prompted the operation may be limited to a specific arterial segment, the intima in the adjacent parent arteries is often loosely attached to the underlying media and vulnerable to detachment. This finding is particularly common in patients with atherosclerotic aneurysmal disease. In patients who have undergone an abdominal aortic aneurysmectomy, postoperative external iliac occlusion from a subintimal dissection beginning at the level of arterial occlusion by a vascular clamp is a recognized, although rare, complication. The use of tourniquets for arterial occlusion is the one method most prone to cause intimal disruption in a patient with atherosclerosis and generally should be avoided.

When arterial clamps are used, they should be applied at an angle least likely to cause intimal fracture or fragmentation. Under ideal circumstances the clamp should be applied to an artery free of grossly palpable atherosclerosis. This is often impossible, and the surgeon must accept some degree of intimal thickening. This is most often encountered in operations for aortic aneurysms in which the common iliac arteries have a greater than normal lumen but have palpable atherosclerotic intimal thickening in a portion of the arterial wall. In this situation, the large arterial lumen indicates that late arterial occlusion is unlikely to occur if a satisfac-

---

[1] Natural latex tubing, $^1/_8$ in. inside diameter, $^1/_{32}$ in. wall thickness. Available from Kent Latex Products, Inc., Kent, Ohio 44240.

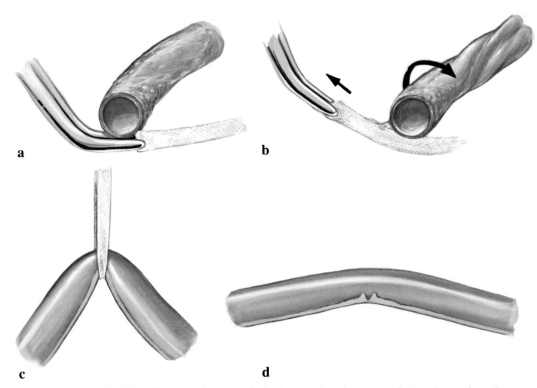

Fig. 2.1,a–d. Fabric sling (**a**, **b**) ensnarls intima and twists vessel; (**c**, **d**) cracks atherosclerotic intima.

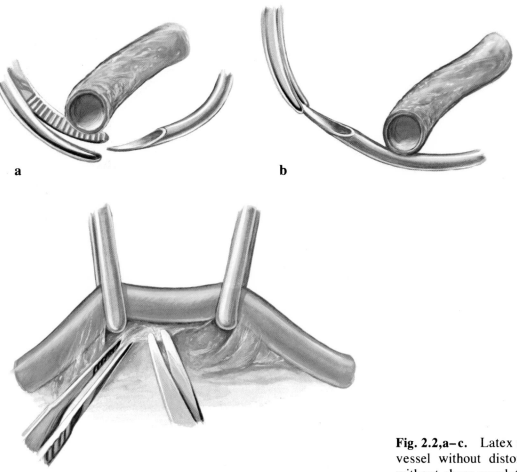

Fig. 2.2,a–c. Latex slings (**a**, **b**) pass around vessel without distortion; (**c**) retract artery without sharp angulation.

11

tory anastomosis has been accomplished, and this location thus may be the preferable site for anastomosis. The arterial clamp on the common iliac artery should be applied to compress the soft portion of the arterial wall against the diseased side (**Fig. 2.3a**). The effect of improper clamp application is illustrated in **Fig. 2.3b.**

Temporary arterial occlusion by means of balloon catheters is occasionally preferable to clamp occlusion. One example occurs when endarterectomy is used to eliminate a short atherosclerotic occlusion in the superficial femoral or popliteal artery. The intima in the patent proximal and distal segments often is thin, friable, and easily detachable. An intraoperative postendarterectomy arteriogram not uncommonly demonstrates a normal lumen in the reconstructed segment but sharp zones of stenosis at the point of application of the arterial clamps, which could have been prevented by the use of balloon catheters passed into the proximal and distal segments.

Two other situations in which balloon catheters are used are illustrated in **Figs. 2.4** and **2.5**. When rapid control of distal backbleeding is required in an operation for rupture of an abdominal aneurysm, or when safe mobilization of the common iliac arteries is difficult to accomplish, insertion of balloon catheters into the iliac orifices accomplishes the desired result (**Fig. 2.4**).

In **Fig. 2.5a** late suture-line disruption of a previous aortofemoral bypass graft has produced a false aneurysm in the groin. Mobilization of the graft and the distal superficial femoral arteries for application of occluding clamps can be easily accomplished. Dissection of the profunda femoris and the posterior branch of the common femoral artery just proximal to it is sometimes difficult and time-consuming. This extensive further dissection can be avoided by incising the false aneurysm and inserting balloon catheters into the orifices of the branch arteries (**Fig. 2.5b**).

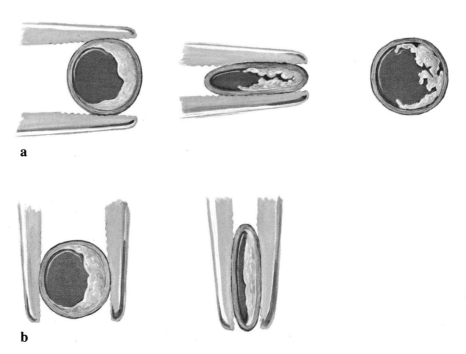

Fig. 2.3,a, b. Clamping an atherosclerotic artery. **a** correct angle; **b** incorrect angle.

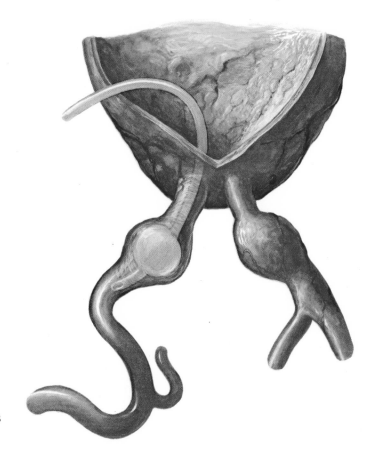

Fig. 2.4. Balloon catheter occlusion of iliac arteries during aortic aneurysmectomy.

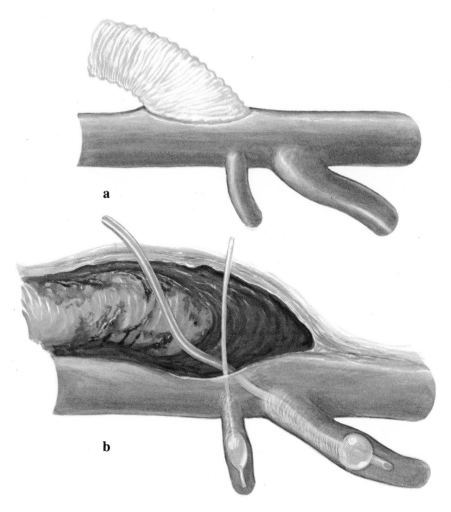

a

b

Fig. 2.5,a, b. Balloon catheter occlusion during false aneurysm repair. **a** original anastomosis; **b** late suture-line disruption and false aneurysm.

Anastomotic and Suture Techniques

In terms of ease of handling and security of knots, silk is our preferred suture material for vascular anastomoses. With continuing stress, however, silk sutures tend to fragment and their use, therefore, is restricted to tissue-

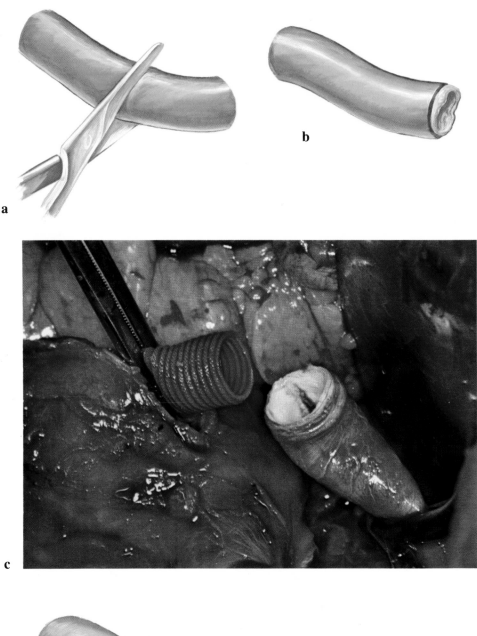

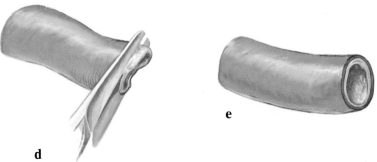

Fig. 2.6. **a, b** retraction of the media after transection of an atherosclerotic artery; **c** operative photograph (note the atherosclerotic rigidity of the intima); **d, e** resection of projecting intima to prepare artery for anastomosis.

to-tissue anastomoses in which the tensile strength of the anastomosis is provided by the cellular connections that develop before the sutures degenerate. Silk sutures are applicable for artery-to-artery, vein-to-vein, or vein-to-artery anastomosis. The long-term integrity of an anastomosis between an artery and a fabric graft depends entirely on the durability of the suture material. Ingrowth of tissue between the artery and the graft to which it is anastomosed is inadequate to maintain tensile strength. A multifilament prosthetic suture retains its strength and in this circumstance is preferred.

In most operations requiring transection of an artery in preparation for a graft anastomosis, one, of course, would attempt to select a level for arterial transection that was free of gross intimal disease, but this is not always feasible. **Fig. 2.6a–c** illustrates the retraction of the media from the rigid intimal core when an atherosclerotic artery is transected. Failure to recognize the retraction of the media may lead the surgeon to place the anastomotic sutures into only the intimal cuff. This error can be avoided by cutting away the projecting intima (**Fig. 2.6d and e**).

Selection of the most appropriate suture techniques in vascular reconstruction depends upon the type of closure required. End-to-end anastomoses between artery-to-artery or artery-to-vein should always be made with interrupted sutures. Dissected or resected vascular segments tend to be constricted by spasm, and even after instrumental dilatation, it is difficult to estimate the eventual diameter that the vessels will assume after blood flow has been restored. If a continuous suture is used, the circumference of the artery or vein at the site of anastomosis will be restricted to the length of the suture, whereas interrupted sutures permit expansion to normal size. **Fig. 2.7a and b** illustrates the stenosis that may be produced by a continuous suture and the prevention of stenosis by the use of interrupted sutures.

This basic principle reappears in numerous situations. Inadvertent lacerations of the arterial wall or actual avulsion of a portion of artery, as illustrated in **Fig. 2.8a and b,** require repair. *Closure* with transverse or figure-of-eight sutures results in arterial constriction whereas interrupted sutures applied in the long axis of the artery preserve arterial size (**Fig. 2.8c–e**). A comparable situation exists with the use of interrupted mattress sutures (**Fig. 2.9**). The formerly held concept that arterial eversion is required

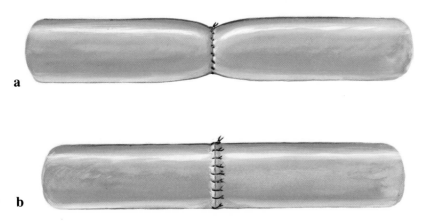

Fig. 2.7,a, b. Suture techniques for end-to-end anastomoses between arteries or veins. **a** stenosis from continuous suture; **b** interrupted sutures allow vessel to expand to normal size.

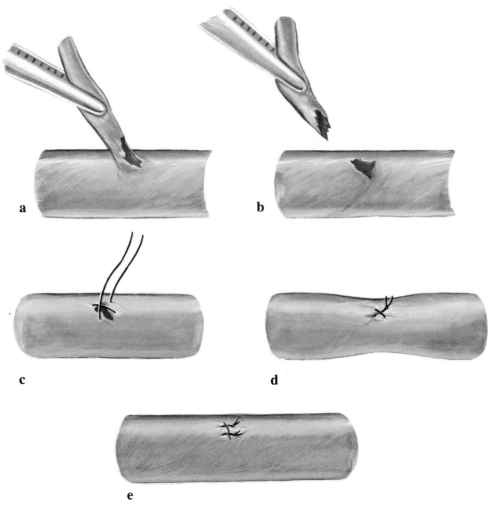

Fig. 2.8, a–e. Suture of arterial or venous tears. **a** avulsion of branch vessel; **b** resulting rent; **c** closure with figure-of-eight suture; **d** resulting stenosis; **e** closure with interrupted simple vertical sutures.

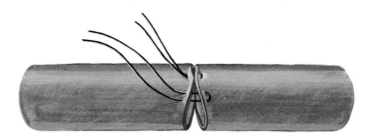

Fig. 2.9. Arterial stenosis from interrupted mattress sutures.

for a satisfactory anastomosis originally prompted the use of mattress sutures. As each stitch is knotted, the enclosed tissue is compressed. Although the degree of resulting stenosis is less than in the instances cited above, it is impossible to prevent some degree of arterial narrowing. Arterial eversion as a mandatory requirement for vascular anastomoses has not been supported in practical application.

The closure of longitudinal arteriotomies or venotomies is most easily performed with continuous sutures. Some degree of constriction of the vessel is inevitable depending upon the depth of the suture bites. The deleterious effect is inversely proportional to the size of the vessel. Thus the narrowing following closure of a longitudinal incision in the aorta is of little importance compared to the luminal constriction following closure of a longitudinal profunda femoris arteriotomy. Whenever arterial narrowing may reduce the effectiveness of the operation, the closure should be supplemented by a patch graft. **Fig. 2.10a and b** illustrates the comparison of simple closure with patch graft closure.

Other considerations, however, may indicate the preferred technique. Simple closure of a longitudinal arteriotomy in the internal carotid artery beyond the end of the carotid bulb is preferred to patch graft closure in order to lessen the time period of cerebral ischemia. In this case, closely spaced sutures that seize no more than 1 mm of arterial wall are used. Aortoiliac endarterectomy, although a generally durable operation, has a small but predictable frequency of late obstructive atherosclerosis. In order to minimize or delay the effect of recurrent atherosclerosis, longitudinal iliac arteriotomies are avoided and the iliac portions of the operations are performed with an arterial stripper passed through transverse arteriotomies. The customary dilatation of the endarterectomized iliac artery has not been lessened as it would have been by closure of a longitudinal arteriotomy, and if atherosclerosis were to reappear, a longer time would pass before restenosis were to develop.

The most commonly used material for patch grafts is the saphenous vein. The portion of the saphenous vein at the level of the ankle is easily accessible. Its size is adequate for most needs and its removal is preferable to the resection of a vein segment in the thigh, which may be needed for venous return in the event the patient were later to develop deep thrombophlebitis. It should not be used in patients with severe ischemia of the lower extremity when healing of a skin incision at this level may be compromised. The patch should be trimmed at each end to produce a narrow but squared end. Separate sutures are applied at each corner of the square **(Fig. 2.11a and b)**.

Trimming the graft to a point or continuing a single suture around the apex carries the same threat of local arterial stenosis that is present when a continuous suture is used to close a transverse arteriotomy. A common mistake is to overestimate the desired width of the patch. It is rarely necessary to use more than a longitudinal half of the vein segment. A wider patch results in a bulge susceptible to mural thrombosis or eventual aneurysmal degeneration **(Fig. 2.12a and b)**. In a few circumstances deliber-

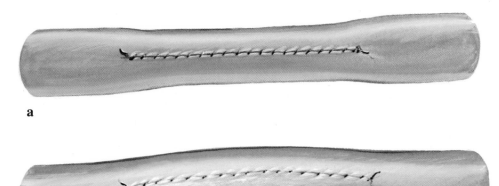

a

b

Fig. 2.10,a, b.   Longitudinal arteriotomy closure. **a** stenosis from simple closure; **b** prevention of stenosis by the use of a patch.

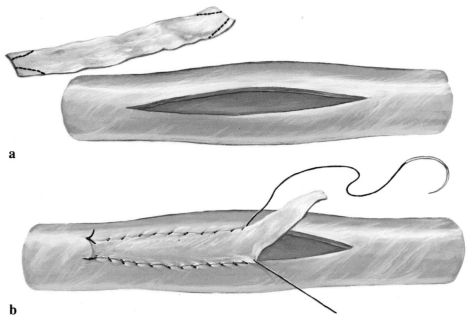

Fig. 2.11,a, b. Preparation and suture of patch grafts. **a** "squaring off" the ends of the patch; **b** interrupted sutures at the apices.

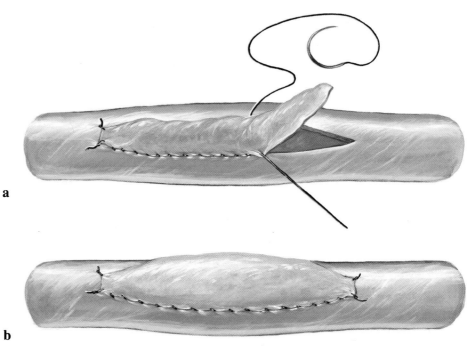

Fig. 2.12,a, b. Width of patch graft. **a** excessively wide venous patch; **b** aneurysmal bulge.

ate abnormal dilatation may be desirable, as in the rare patient who develops early arterial stenosis secondary to fibroplasia following carotid endarterectomy. A wide patch graft after a second endarterectomy may delay the influence of a subsequent fibroplastic reaction. Another instance occurs in the patient who has undergone a local endarterectomy in the popliteal artery. Some degree of intimal thickening will usually be present at the distal end point. Tack-down sutures secure the distal intima in place and a patch graft extending beyond the end point tends to contour the flow of blood over the distal ridge and reduce the possibility of thrombosis as a result of turbulence at this point (**Fig. 2.13a and b**).

End-to-end anastomoses between small arteries, or small vein-to-artery grafts, depend upon precise placement of interrupted 6–0 or 7–0 sutures. The potential for error is reduced if the ends of the vessels to be united are spatulated (**Fig. 2.14a and b**). The distance from the apex to the tip should be the same for each segment. This permits the use of a continuous suture along the sides of the anastomosis without threat of resulting stenosis so long as the ends are squared and the suture is interrupted at each end.

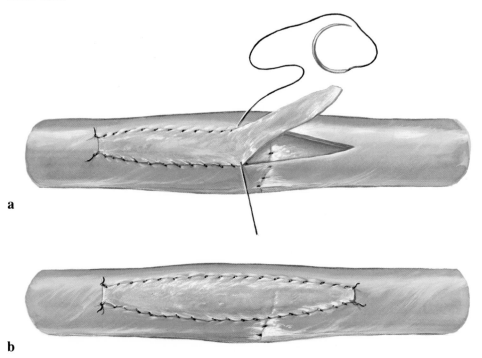

a

b

Fig. 2.13,a, b. Patch supplement to endarterectomy. **a** The arteriotomy is extended beyond the endarterectomy end point, which has been secured with tackdown sutures. **b** Completed patch.

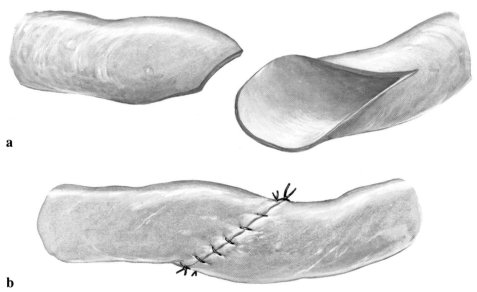

a

b

Fig. 2.14,a, b. Spatulation for small vessel anastomoses. **a** spatulated arterial ends; **b** completed anastomosis.

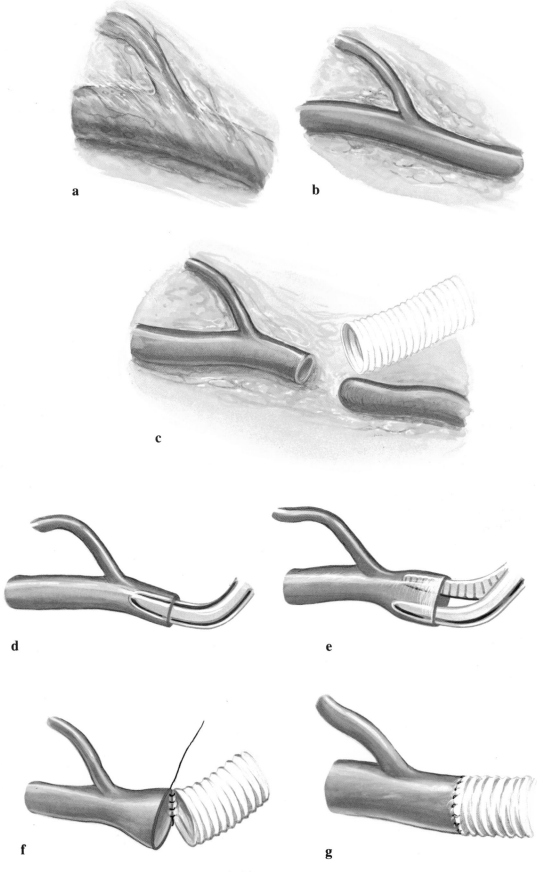

Fig. 2.15,a–g. Anastomosis in presence of arterial spasm. **a** arterial size before mobilization; **b** arterial size after mobilization; **c** resulting graft-artery size difference; **d, e** instrumental dilatation of artery; **f, g** anastomosis performed.

Dissection of small arteries, e.g., renal or profunda femoris, in preparation for establishing an arterial graft inevitably produces spasm and marked reduction in size. **Fig. 2.15a and b** illustrates the degree of narrowing that develops after skeletonization of such an artery. **Fig. 2.15c** illustrates the problem that appears when a graft of appropriate size is brought in approximation to the constricted artery to which it is to be anastomosed. Stretching by the spreading of the jaws of hemostat within the artery will temporarily overcome spasm (**Fig. 2.15d and e**). The anastomosis can then be completed with accurate alignment of the sutures (**Fig. 2.15f and g**). Continuous sutures are usually appropriate for an end-to-end anastomosis between the conventional fabric graft and a large artery. The rigidity of the graft tends to prevent the purse-stringing effect that is more likely to occur when an autogenous tissue graft is used. Interrupted sutures are preferred for smaller synthetic grafts (5–6 mm) when these are used for small artery anastomoses, e.g., renal or profunda femoris arteries.

In operations performed for atherosclerotic disease it would be desirable that all anastomoses were made to arterial segments free of disease, but this opportunity rarely exists. For this reason the suturing techniques should be adapted to the local pathology. Insertion of the suture from outside the artery into its lumen may separate the loosely attached intima (**Fig. 2.16a**). Other things being equal, the preferred technique is to pass sutures on the arterial side of the anastomosis from inside to out (**Fig. 2.16b**).

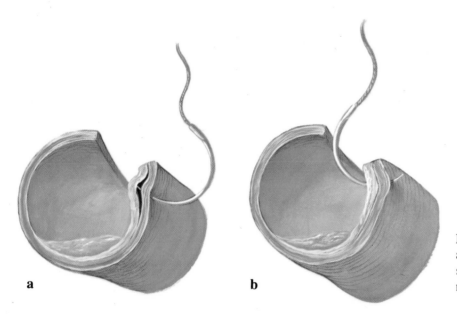

a   b

Fig. 2.16,a, b. Insertion of sutures in atherosclerotic arteries. **a** intimal separation from external insertion of needle; **b** internal insertion of needle.

When grasping the arterial wall with a forceps particular care should be taken to prevent instrumental disruption of the intima or a lateral tear in the arterial wall (**Fig. 2.17a**). In situations where it is necessary to insert the suture from the outside, one can use the forceps as a stabilizing counterpressure tool. They should be held against the arterial wall from inside as the needle is inserted from the outside (**Fig. 2.17b**).

Often it becomes necessary to anastomose a graft to an artery in which the intima may have areas of calcification impervious to the insertion of the suture needle; this occasionally happens when the iliac arm of a graft in an aortic aneurysm operation is to be sutured to the end of a divided common iliac artery. The arterial lumen is usually slightly larger than normal and thus is a satisfactory outflow vessel. Penetration of the calcified portion of the circumference for insertion of the anastomotic sutures

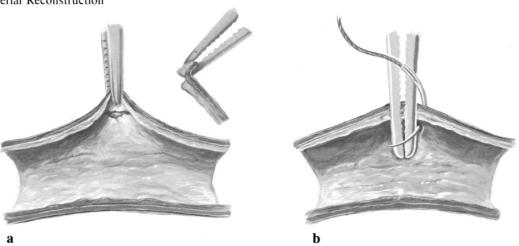

Fig. 2.17,a, b. Forceps and the atherosclerotic artery. **a** intimal tear; **b** closed-forceps technique.

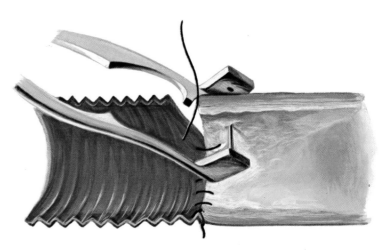

Fig. 2.18. Arterial punch in sclerotic artery.

may be made with an arterial punch without disrupting the arterial wall or fracturing the plaque (**Fig. 2.18**).

An end-to-end anastomosis between artery and graft is often complicated by disparity in size between graft and artery. This can be overcome by wider spacing of the sutures on the side with the greater circumference. This technique should be restricted to those portions of the arterial wall that retain normal pliability. When a portion of the arterial wall contains an atheromatous plaque, sutures in this portion of the arterial wall should be aligned accurately to the graft. Failure to do so results in anastomotic leakage that is difficult to control with additional sutures. **Fig. 2.19a–d** illustrates the common circumstance where the posterior wall of the artery has been infiltrated with a rigid atheroma. The "make-up" sutures are restricted to the anterior two-thirds of the anastomosis.

After completion of an anastomosis and release of the occluding clamps, bleeding is often observed from needle holes or in gaps between the sutures. Minor openings where the jet of blood is comparable in size to that from a 22-gauge needle will generally seal off spontaneously. This can be hastened by temporary reapplication of the clamps or by holding the gloved finger over the opening until bleeding stops. Larger openings require additional sutures (**Fig. 2.20a**). Placement of additional sutures after the clamps have been removed often causes longitudinal tears in the artery as the sutures are tied (**Fig. 2.20b**). The preferred technique is to reapply and approximate the clamps so that the suture may be secured without tension (**Fig. 2.20c and d**).

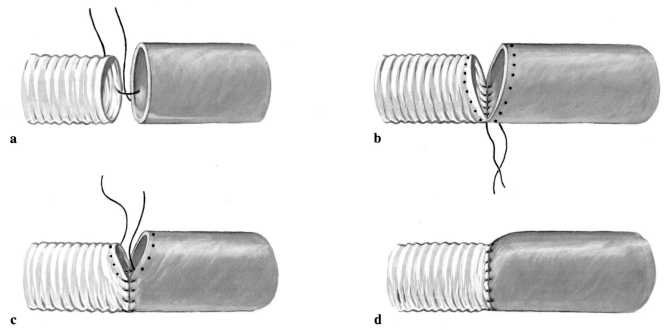

Fig. 2.19,a–d. Disparity in graft-artery size when the atherosclerotic plaque is confined to a segment of the arterial circumference. **a, b** evenly spaced sutures in diseased segment; **c, d** unevenly spaced sutures in the undiseased segment.

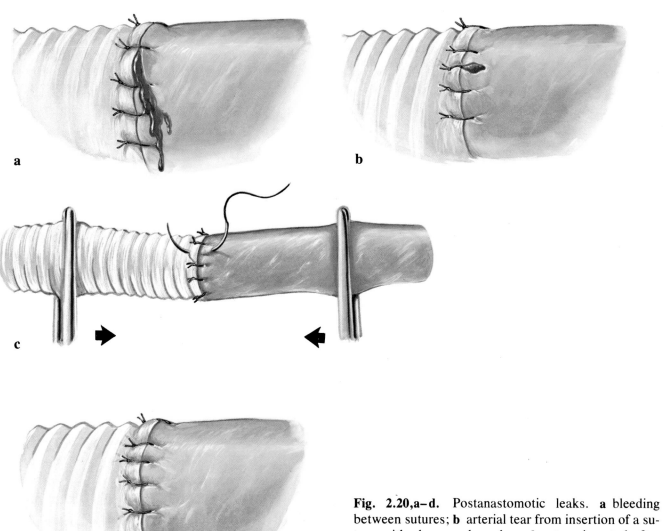

Fig. 2.20,a–d. Postanastomotic leaks. **a** bleeding between sutures; **b** arterial tear from insertion of a suture with clamps released; **c, d** suture inserted after reapplication of clamps.

23

Large tears in the arterial wall may be difficult to close with simple sutures without causing gross distortion of the arterial lumen. This problem most commonly occurs during careless closure of an endarterectomized artery when the sutures are pulled too tightly or a lateral tear is created by rough use of the forceps (**Fig. 2.21a**); occasionally it is encountered during endarterectomy when the dissecting instrument inadvertently penetrates the full thickness of the arterial wall. An attempt to use one or more vertical sutures to close the defect often results in widening of the defect as a result of sutures tearing through the arterial wall. Deeply placed transverse sutures may narrow the arterial lumen. The remedy is the application of a multitude of "darn" sutures using 6–0 thread (**Fig. 2.21b**). Each suture is loosely placed and set into position without tension, and this technique in essence creates a fabric patch that is secured to the artery at multiple points around its circumference. This type of suture would be used to close the tear shown in Fig. 2.20b.

A simple oblique transection of a graft to be used for an end-to-side anastomosis creates the hazard of developing a short zone of arterial constriction at the apex of the graft unless extreme care is used in the shallow placement of sutures adjacent to the apex (**Fig. 2.22a and b**). The effect is comparable to the closure of a longitudinal arteriotomy. This problem is overcome by squaring off the ends of the graft (**Fig. 2.23a**). This tends to spread the "V" at the apex of the arteriotomy and creates the same effect as closure of a transverse arteriotomy at that point (**Fig. 2.23b and c**). One can then use deeper sutures at the end of the graft without concern for producing stenosis in the recipient artery.

One is often tempted to remove an ellipse from the wall of the recipient vessel when an end-to-side anastomosis is being created. This has some validity in vein-to-vein anastomosis, e.g., portal decompression operations, where the intravenous pressure may be insufficient to spread the

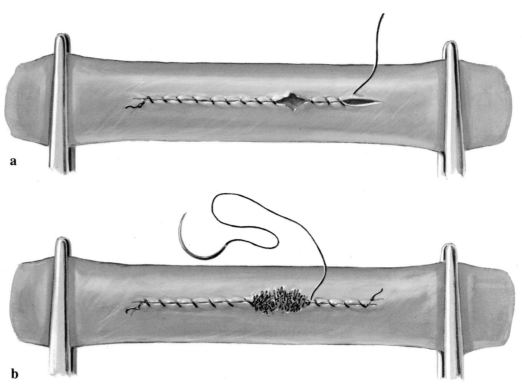

Fig. 2.21,a, b. Closure of vents or tears with darn sutures. **a** arterial defect; **b** darn sutures.

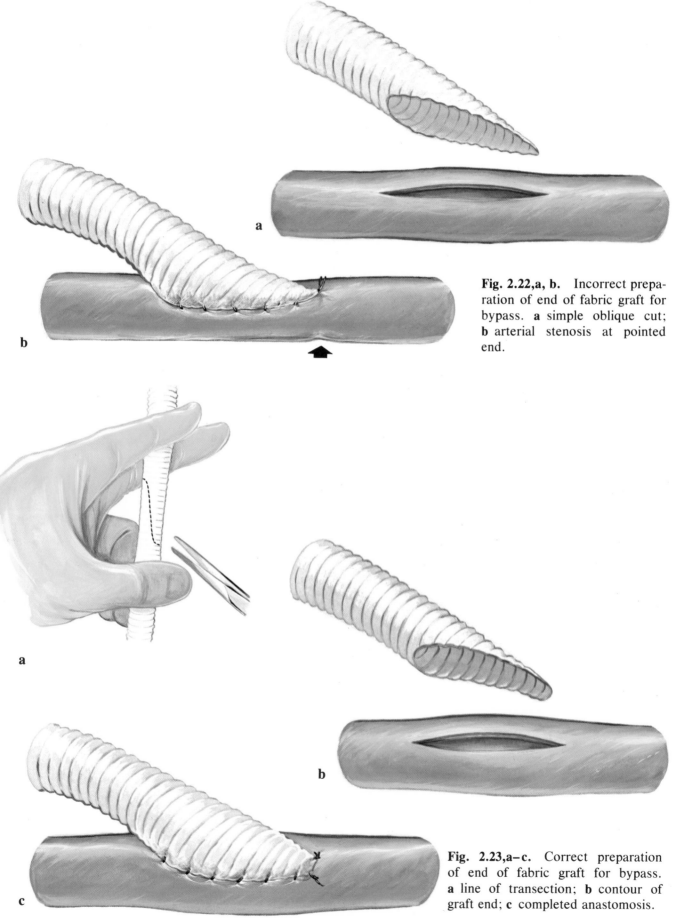

Fig. 2.22,a, b. Incorrect preparation of end of fabric graft for bypass. **a** simple oblique cut; **b** arterial stenosis at pointed end.

Fig. 2.23,a–c. Correct preparation of end of fabric graft for bypass. **a** line of transection; **b** contour of graft end; **c** completed anastomosis.

25

stoma to its widest possible dimension. In the high-pressure arterial system, an adequate stoma will develop with the use of a simple longitudinal arteriotomy in the recipient vessel (**Fig. 2.24a–c**). With an elliptical incision, the spreading of the remaining arterial wall flattens the central portion of the graft (**Fig. 2.25a–c**). The entry point for blood flow is thus at the proximal end of the anastomosis and unless extreme care is used in placing the sutures in the proximal apex, stenosis of the graft may occur at that point. In extreme situations, the posterior wall of the recipient artery will be drawn anteriorly, thereby flattening the arterial lumen at the very point where a large and well-shaped lumen is most desirable (**Fig. 2.25d**).

A pertinent clinical situation is present in the patient who needs an aortofemoral bypass operation. A mild degree of atherosclerotic thickening is often present in the posterior common femoral intima. The desired anastomosis is one made to a simple arteriotomy that extends to a point just beyond the end of the atheroma. The arterial lumen at the site of anastomosis becomes increased as a result of the increase in circumference that the graft adds to the artery. Encroachment of the lumen by further growth of the atheroma is unlikely to be hemodynamically significant. Resection of a portion of the arterial wall by an elliptical incision reduces the graft-artery circumference. Lateral distention of the graft when blood flow is restored flattens the posterior wall of the artery. This brings the atheroma in closer approximation to the anterior surface of the graft, thereby increasing the potential for occlusion as the atheroma thickens.

Fig. 2.26a–c illustrates two methods for creating an end-to-side anastomosis between a graft and a major artery (usually the aorta). The technique shown in **Fig. 22.6a and b** encloses a portion of the arterial wall within the jaws of a partially occluding clamp. The purpose of this technique is to preserve blood flow in the artery. Except for graft anastomosis to the ascending aorta to bypass an innominate artery lesion, there are few circumstances in the operations to be described where complete inter-

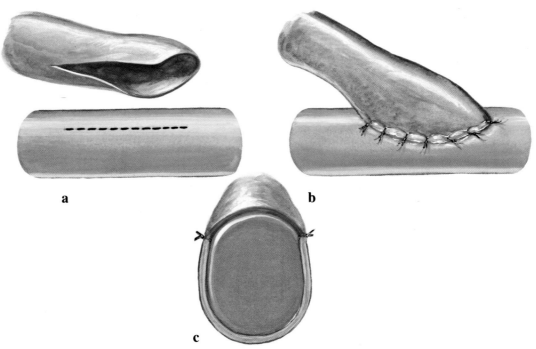

Fig. 2.24,a–c. Anastomosis of a vein graft to a simple longitudinal arteriotomy. **a** "cobra hood" shape of graft end; **b** ideal contour of completed anastomosis; **c** cross section.

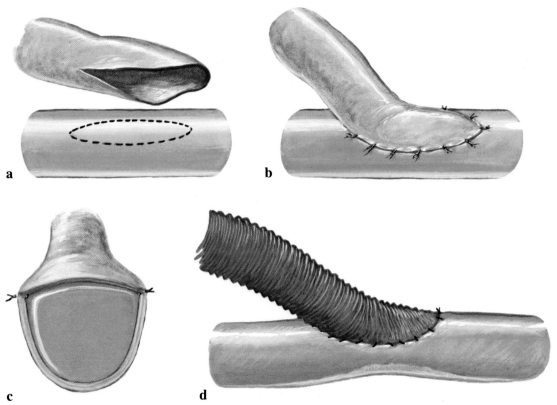

Fig. 2.25,a–d. Anastomosis of a vein graft to an elliptical arteriotomy. **a** elliptical arteriotomy; **b** flattened graft with restricted stoma; **c** cross section; **d** posterior arterial wall pulled into stoma.

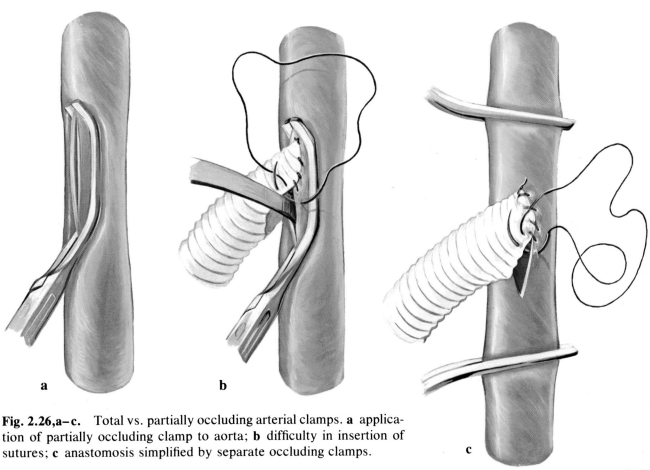

Fig. 2.26,a–c. Total vs. partially occluding arterial clamps. **a** application of partially occluding clamp to aorta; **b** difficulty in insertion of sutures; **c** anastomosis simplified by separate occluding clamps.

27

ruption of blood flow is not tolerated in the time interval required for completion of an anastomosis. The disadvantages of this technique appear most notably in the situation where it is most commonly used: anastomosing the aortic segment of a bifurcated dacron graft to the side of the infrarenal aorta. The lateral surfaces of the aorta are compressed against one another. Unless one places the sutures close to the edge of the aorta, a technique not advised for this anastomosis in a diseased aortic wall, it is difficult to avoid inclusion of the opposite side of the aorta within the sutures. Furthermore, the intima of the aorta is usually grossly diseased with atherosclerosis and is vulnerable to disruption and fragmentation at the site of application of the partially occluding clamp. Unless one applies an additional completely occluding clamp when the flushing maneuvers are performed, intimal fragments may be swept away to lodge in the distal arterial tree after release of the partially occluding clamp.

Fig. 2.26c illustrates the preferred technique. Totally occluding clamps are placed proximal and distal to the aortotomy. The sides of the aorta tend to open widely, and loose debris within the aorta can be flushed or irrigated free. Each suture may be applied deeply into the wall of the aorta under clear vision and away from the opposite arterial wall. The final flushing maneuvers can be performed by alternate release of the distal and proximal clamps before forward blood flow through the aorta is restored.

Fig. 2.27a and b illustrates the useful technique for anastomosing a tubular fabric graft to the side of the aorta when a small graft is necessary to match the size of the artery to which it is to be connected distally. One example is an aorta-to-celiac graft where a 6-mm graft is the appropriate size. The graft is cut from a 12 × 6 bifurcation graft preserving a flange of its aortic segment. The flange allows for the rapid placement of deep sutures in the aortic wall without the risk of narrowing the stoma.

Placement of aortorenal grafts in patients with renal artery atherosclerosis is a common revascularization technique. The wall of the aorta is usually thickened by atherosclerosis. A 5-mm tubular graft that conforms

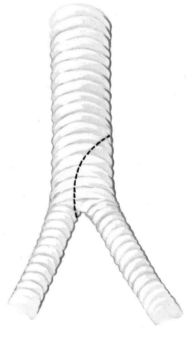
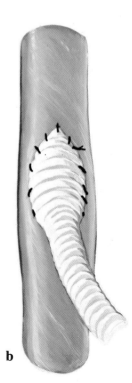

Fig. 2.27, a, b. Flanged fabric grafts. a method of preparation; b appearance of anastomosis. 	a	b

to the size of the outflow artery is often difficult to anastomose to the aorta. The procedure is simplified by using a flanged graft cut from a 10 × 5 bifurcation graft. A generous ellipse can be removed from the aortic wall. A flange of greater dimension than the one shown (**Fig. 2.27**) is created by including more of the contralateral iliac and aortic fabric to match the dimensions of the opening in the aorta. When sutured in place the flange becomes, in effect, a patch on the aorta with a graft emerging from its center. The sutures are easy to apply and the suture line is removed from the zone of turbulence at the point of exit of the graft.

Endarterectomy

The various techniques for performing endarterectomy are described in connection with specific operations, but certain general comments are appropriate for inclusion in this section. Endarterectomy can be performed only in arteries in which atherosclerosis has produced cleavage planes in the arterial wall. The correct cleavage plane for endarterectomy is illustrated in **Fig. 2.28a and b.** Pathologic sections of the specimen with appro-

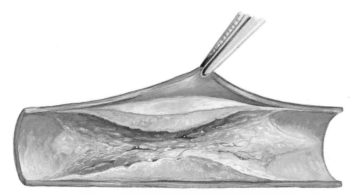

a

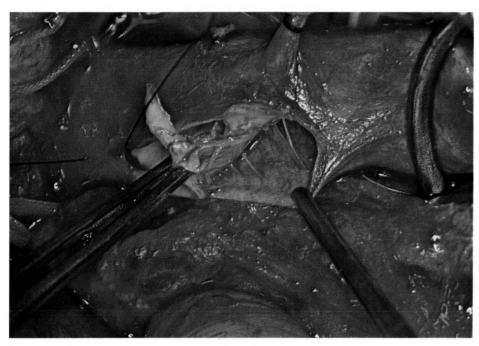

b

Fig. 2.28. a The usually preferred tissue plane for endarterectomy. **b** Endarterectomy in progress. Note the color of the inner surface of the portion of the artery where the intima has been partially removed. Tissue tags between the specimen and the arterial wall will need to be picked away before the arteriotomy is closed.

priate staining discloses atherosclerotic intima and a thin layer of the innermost fibers of the media. In this plane the dissecting instrument encounters little or no resistance. The surface of the residual media is smooth and has the brownish-red color of muscle tissue. A more shallow plane entirely within the intimal layer is usually equally simple to dissect (**Fig. 2.29a and b**). The inner surface of the residual arterial wall has the pale yellow hue of an atheroma. Endarterectomy in this plane may invite the early recurrence of luminal obstruction. **Fig. 2.30** illustrates a deep subadventitial dissection plane. Dissection in this plane is met with resistance, and the inner surface of the arterial wall is ragged and thin and susceptible to disruption.

The ideal distal endarterectomy end point is at a point where the atheromatous lesion comes to an abrupt end. In the most favorable situation the atheroma usually ends in a tapered point. The intima bordering the point and beyond will be normally adherent to the underlying media. As the dissection plane is developed in the customary plane, the final event is the separation of the distal tongue of intima from its connection with the adjacent intima. At this point, the actual endarterectomy becomes confined to the small portion of the arterial circumference containing the atheroma. The thinly feathered edges at the point of the resected specimen usually indicates the accomplishment of an adequate end point at which the residual intima is firmly attached.

Not all atheromatous lesions provide this favorable situation. The arteriographic appearance of short occlusive lesions in the popliteal artery may suggest a normal artery beyond the occlusion. The intima in this portion is almost invariably thickened to a slight degree and is easily separable. An open endarterectomy is an ideal operation for this lesion. The development of the end point requires circumferential transection of the intima beyond the obstructing lesions, tack-down sutures at the end point and closure with a vein patch.

In another variant of atherosclerosis the intima adjacent to and beyond the distal tongue of atheroma may be only loosely attached to the subjacent media. Distal projection of the dissecting instrument in the original cleavage plane continues to separate the arterial wall beyond the end of the atheroma. This is not uncommon during carotid endarterectomy. If one recognizes that this is about to occur, the dissection plane can often be altered to a slightly more superficial level as the end point is approached.

The awareness of this variant is particularly important in the performance of the various semi-closed eversion endarterectomy operations for obstructing lesions at the arterial orifice in which the endarterectomy is performed through an arteriotomy in the parent artery. This variant is often encountered in atherosclerosis of the renal, superior mesenteric, and celiac arteries. Its presence can be suspected if the preoperative arteriograms show a pattern of slight but generalized dilatation or ectasia of the aorta and its branching arteries. It can also be suspected whenever the aortic intima when first separated at the beginning of the endarterectomy presents as a thick but soft, pliable, rubbery layer extending to the orifice of the branch artery. The recognition is certain later in the operation if the distal dissection in the wall of the prolapsing branch artery yields a thin walled cylinder of intima still attached distally and longer than the obstructing lesion. If this occurs, the cylinder should be transected at the distal level of the dissection. Although the end point will no longer be visible after the prolapse is reduced, it must be assumed that a distal flap remains and that corrective steps must be taken. One may make the same assumption whenever the endarterectomy specimen breaks free spontaneously but has a cylinder of thin intima at its distal end.

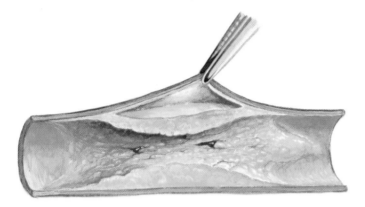

a

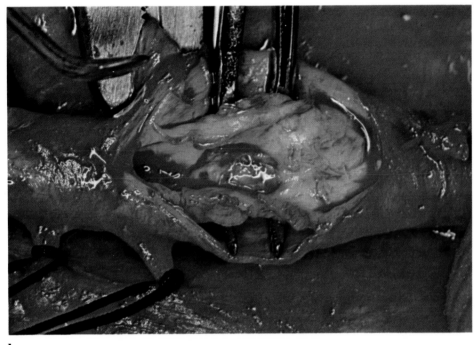

b

Fig. 2.29. **a** A shallow, and incorrect, endarterectomy plane. **b** Demonstration of two potential endarterectomy planes by passage of a clamp behind a central core of atheroma. The plane at the top is the preferred one in most situations. The plane at the bottom has been developed within the atheromatous intima.

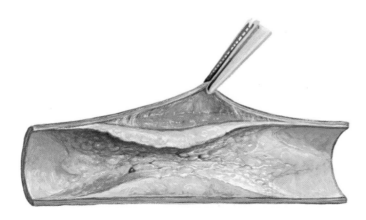

Fig. 2.30. A deep, and incorrect, subadventitial endarterectomy plane.

31

In the more common form of atherosclerosis in the branch arteries of the aorta, the lesion ends in the tapered point described above. This can be anticipated when endarterectomy in the aortic portion of the operation yields a densely sclerotic and rigid intima. Renal dissection in the customary endarterectomy plane usually terminates at a satisfactory end point as the specimen breaks free.

Eversion endarterectomy is a commonly applied in situ technique for removing atherosclerotic orifice lesions in the vertebral, visceral, and renal arteries. It is also particularly valuable for obtaining an autogenous tissue artery graft to be used in places where a fabric graft would be unsuitable, i.e., in areas of infection. An occluded superficial femoral artery is the most frequently used donor vessel. **Fig. 2.31a–c** illustrates the steps in preparing the resected occluded segment. The smooth dissection plane described above is difficult to develop in this artery. The surgeon will usually observe scattered areas where the deeper layers of the intima remain firmly attached. Scraping the surface of the everted artery with a scalpel is often necessary to create a smooth surface. To reduce the eversion a small arterial stripper is inserted, its ring sutured to the distal end and then withdrawn.

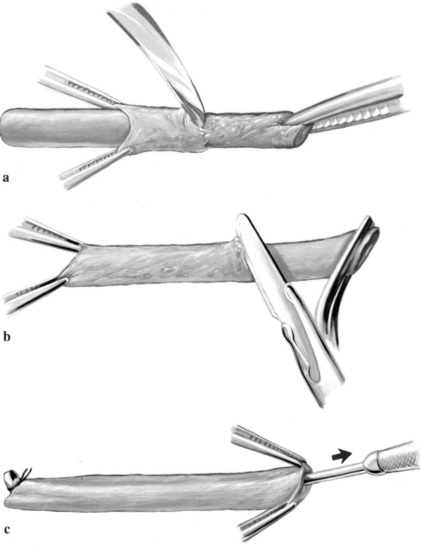

Fig. 2.31,a–c. Eversion endarterectomy. **a** endarterectomy in progress; **b** removal of residual intimal plaque; **c** reduction of eversion by use of a small arterial stripper.

The four photographs in **Fig. 2.32a–d** illustrate from dog experiments the gross appearance of the lumen of an endarterectomized artery in four stages of healing and intimal regeneration.

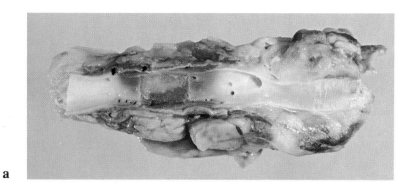

a

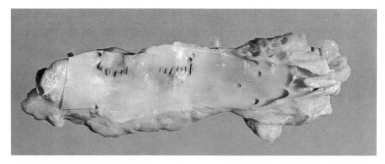

b

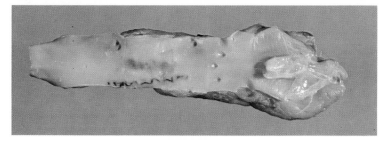

c

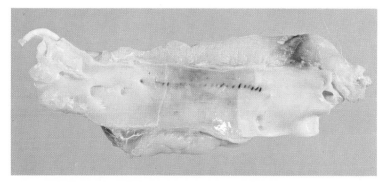

d

Fig. 2.32,a–d. Photographs of the luminal surface of a canine aorta after excision of a 1-cm segment of the inner lining including the intima and a portion of the media. At four days the defect has been filled by a layer of unorganized thrombus. Subendothelial hemorrhage can be seen adjacent to the zone of excision (**a**). The progression at 3 weeks (**b**), 6 months (**c**), and 8 months (**d**) results in replacement of the thrombus by a glistening layer of pale tissue that fills in the defect.

Microscopically the leukocytes in the layer of thrombus become at first pyknotic and then seemingly convert in situ into fibroblasts. These become longitudinally oriented and the surface cells flatten to resemble the shape of normal endothelium. Elastic tissue is notably absent. The regenerative process appears to be completed at 8 months.

Operative Arteriograms

Operative arteriograms at the time of the procedure are obtained in many arterial reconstructive operations in which small arteries have been clamped, anastomosed, or endarterectomized. These have become a routine in renal artery operations and reconstructive procedures distal to the common femoral arteries. The film may disclose unanticipated gross defects at the suture lines or at the point of application of occluding clamps that require correction.

Platelet Aggregation

Adenosine diphosphate (ADP) release at the site of intimal injury encourages the local accumulation of platelets, a normal mechanism that helps in sealing suture lines. In patients with platelet hyperaggregatability, platelet accumulation at the point of anastomosis can produce immediate and substantial stenosis of the artery. This is of little significance in major arteries with a large volume of blood flow. In smaller arteries such as the renal, or the profunda and superficial femoral arteries, severe stenosis or even early occlusion may develop (**Fig. 2.33a and b**). This phenomenon usually develops within the first few moments of restoration of blood flow. When it is discovered, revision of the anastomosis is required, occasionally with enlargement of the stoma with a patch graft. The demonstration of an amorphous, friable, gray mass at the suture line confirms the diagnosis. In one patient, restenosis of an aorta-arterial autograft anastomosis for renal artery repair appeared four times and was finally overcome only after numerous units of banked blood (platelet-deficient after 24 hours of storage) were infused to restore blood lost during the repeated operations. An aspirin/persantine regimen is probably advisable in these patients for the first few postoperative weeks.[1]

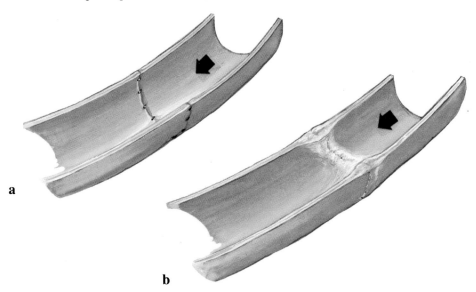

a

b

Fig. 2.33,a, b. Platelet accumulation on suture line. **a** suture line; **b** platelet accumulation with resulting stenosis.

---

[1] Platelet dysfunction may occur in which bleeding, not clotting, is the problem. Blood replacement by banked blood is necessary in most major arterial operations. The platelet activity in banked blood is rapidly lost when blood replacement in excess of 2500 ml is required—and clotting deficiencies become apparent. The infusion of preserved platelets (10 packs) and fresh frozen plasma (2 units) aids in overcoming the deficit.

Clamp Defects

The arteriogram may disclose a short zone of stenosis that is caused by disruption of the arterial intima at the point of clamp application to the artery in patients with atherosclerosis. This is most commonly seen in the superficial femoral and popliteal arteries. Correction is required and since vulnerability to clamp occlusion has been demonstrated, balloon catheters should be used for proximal and distal control rather than reapplication of arterial clamps.

Another type of clamp defect may occur in small arteries, often in segments without obvious atherosclerosis. In this, the intimal surfaces of the two sides of the artery at the site of the clamp tend to adhere to one another after clamp release. This is usually, but not always, visible when one inspects the exterior of the artery (**Fig. 2.34a and b**). The vertebral artery, the renal artery and its terminal branches, the inferior mesenteric artery, and the profunda femoris and its lateral and terminal branches are particularly susceptible to this defect. Less so is the internal carotid artery distal to the carotid bulb, but one should suspect the presence of a clamp defect if less than the anticipated backflow occurs after release of the distal clamp.

The defect is overcome by passage of an arterial dilator of appropriate size (2 mm in profunda branches, 4 mm in the carotid artery). It is important to avoid reapplication of clamps. **Fig. 2.35a and b** illustrates a hypothetical situation in which a dilator is being passed before the application of the final sutures in a venous patch graft. Backbleeding is then controlled by digital pressure or the insertion of a balloon catheter during completion of the suture line. This phenomenon only rarely occurs in an endarterectomized artery. Thus if one were performing an extensive profundaplasty with vein patch angioplasty the first sutures of the patch would be applied to the distal end to allow successive removal of the clamps on the distal branches, passage of dilators, and repositioning of the clamp onto the endarterectomized segment.

Thrombosis

Prevention of thrombosis in the distal arterial tree during the time of clamp occlusion of the proximal arteries is an integral part of all arterial operations. This can be accomplished by total body heparinization, but often the

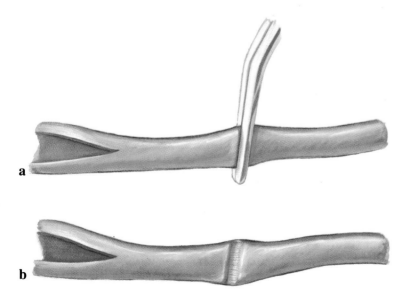

Fig. 2.34,a, b. Arterial stenosis from clamp compression. **a** clamp in place; **b** residual defect.

35

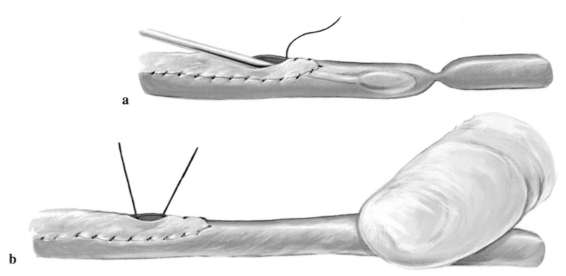

Fig. 2.35,a, b. Correction of clamp defect. **a** arterial dilator; **b** finger compression during completion of suture line.

heparinization introduces a major problem in maintaining hemostasis in the operative area during the various dissection, graft anastomosis, and arteriotomy closure maneuvers.

In most arterial operations, varying degrees of blood flow continue to perfuse the distal arterial tree after a proximal clamp is applied. The adequacy of collateral blood flow in this situation varies in different organ systems and is, of course, modified by the presence or absence of disease in the collateral arteries. The extent of collateral flow can be gauged by observing the volume of backbleeding after release of the distal occluding clamp.

In almost every operation, however, the distal arterial segment adjacent to the occluding clamp is particularly vulnerable to early thrombosis. **Fig. 2.36a** illustrates the flow pattern distal to an arterial clamp. Blood is returning to the distal arterial tree by retrograde flow through normal distal arteries. This could represent the return of flow into the proximal common femoral artery by way of the circumflex iliac and inferior epigastric arteries after clamp occlusion of the proximal external iliac artery. The column of blood between the clamp and the branch artery is static, and intraluminal thrombosis to the level of the branch artery can be expected within 5–15 min (**Fig. 2.36b**). The presence or absence of thrombosis in this segment can be determined by observing the volume of backbleeding after release of the clamp, a maneuver that should be performed repeatedly during any operation (**Fig. 2.36c**).

If backbleeding is sparse or absent, one should suspect that thrombus has accumulated. If thrombosis has just begun, it may often be expressed by forceful compression of soft tissue distally. **Fig. 2.36d** shows forceful thigh compression to eject thrombus in the external iliac artery. If thrombus followed by free bleeding does not appear, the passage of a Fogarty balloon catheter is necessary. If thrombosis has already extended beyond the distal arterial branches, this maneuver may be only partially effective in removing the distal thrombus. Thrombosis to this extent should not occur with appropriate precautions.

Installation of dilute heparin solution in sufficient volume to displace the blood in the blind segment should be done at an early stage in the operation (**Fig. 2.37a**) and repeated each time the clamp is released to assess

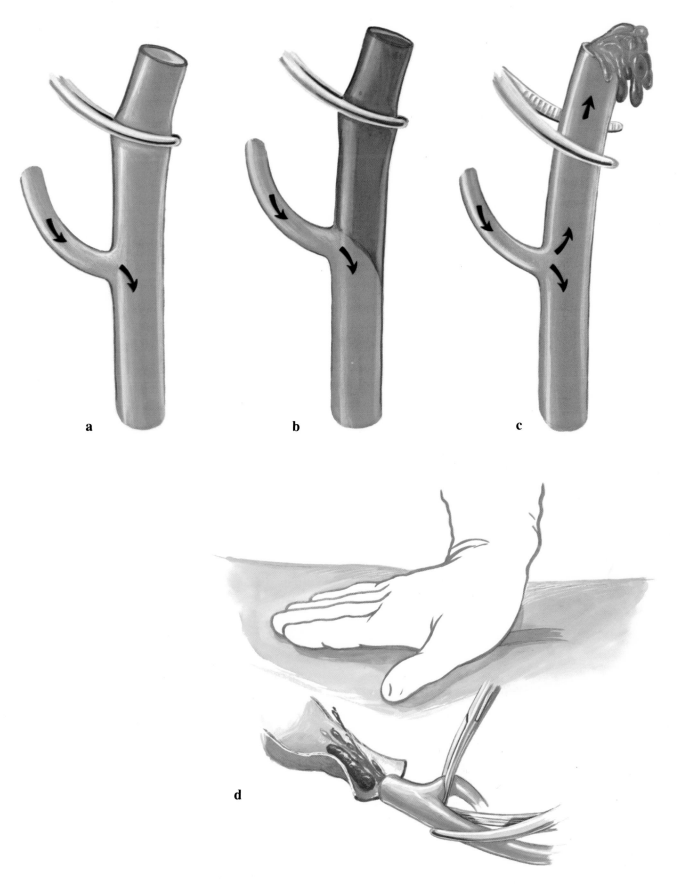

Fig. 2.36,a–d. Distal thrombosis during grafting operations. **a** pattern of blood flow distal to an occluding arterial clamp; **b** thrombus in the blind segment; **c** release of clamp to flush thrombus; **d** compression of thigh to eject attached thrombus.

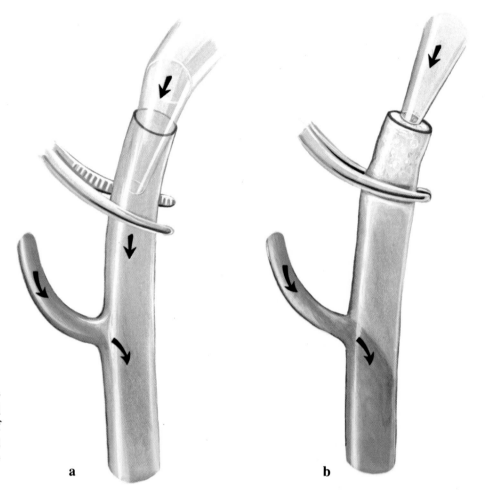

Fig. 2.37,a, b. Local heparinization to prevent distal thrombosis. **a** installation of heparin into blind segment; **b** heparin flush of open arterial stump.

back flow. It is important to recognize that unless a full systemic heparinization dose is given, one cannot adequately heparinize the entire leg for longer than a few minutes, since the venous outflow will quickly remove all of the heparin except for that portion that remains in the static column. The distal arterial tree may remain patent even when clot is present in the static segment, as would be the situation with crossclamping of the subclavian artery where there is a particularly abundant arterial collateral supply to the arm.

In the lower extremities where arterial collateral supply is less, abundant distal thrombosis can usually be anticipated in time and is almost certain to occur if there are multiple distal lesions, which decrease flow even further. For this reason, systemic heparinization is induced once the proximal end of an aortofemoral graft is secure and dry. Introduction of systemic heparinization prior to establishing the proximal anastomosis is preferred by some surgeons but may complicate the procedure if additional suturing becomes necessary in the now awkward to reach posterior aspect of the anastomosis.

In the preceding drawings (Fig. 2.36) there is one area that is even more vulnerable to thrombus accumulation—the arterial stump proximal to the occluding clamp. Blood in this stump, exposed to air, will begin to clot almost immediately during the period of graft anastomosis. Repeated irrigation of this segment with dilute heparin solution is mandatory (**Fig. 2.37b**).

Special precautions are also necessary to prevent thrombotic occlusion of a graft. The preclotting maneuvers illustrated in **Fig. 2.38a and b** are helpful in lessening the period of interstitial graft bleeding once the graft is in place. Blood is instilled into the graft until leakage through the graft ceases. The graft should then be stripped to remove all blood except that which has clotted within the interstices of the graft. When the proximal anastomosis has been completed, the graft is given a final flush with blood to evaluate the adequacy of the suture line. Blood is then stripped from the graft as before and the lumen filled with dilute heparin (**Fig. 2.38c**). Heparin at this time will not lyse the thrombus within the fabric of the graft. A clamp is then applied to the distal segment of the graft to contain the heparin within the graft in preparation for the distal anastomosis. The final maneuver is to assure proximal and distal patency by observing the volume of bleeding during selective release of the proximal and distal clamps before the final sutures are applied.

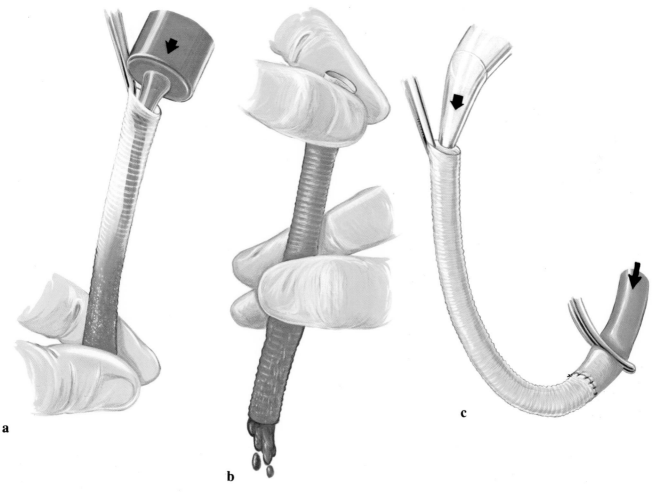

a

b

c

Fig. 2.38,a–c. Prevention of graft thrombosis. **a** preclotting of fabric graft; **b** milking graft to remove intraluminal thrombus; **c** refilling preclotted graft with heparin.

39

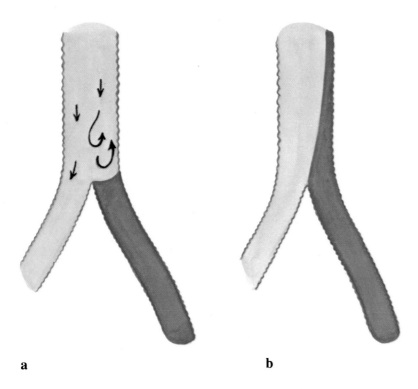

a

b

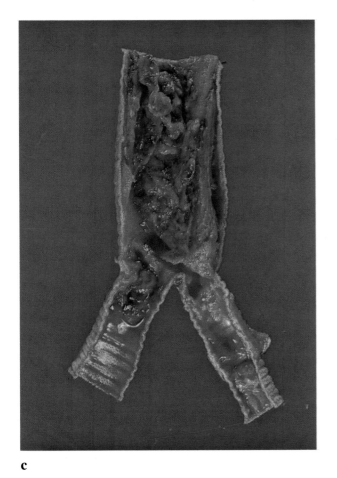

c

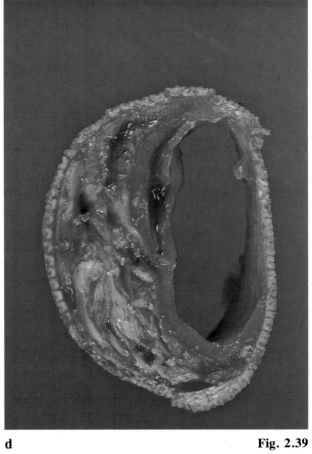

d

Fig. 2.39

Graft Size

Selection of the most appropriate graft size may be a critical decision, particularly for bypass operations. Blood flow through a normal artery is laminar in the sense that flow velocity is most rapid in the center of the artery and decreases as it approaches the intimal surface. This differential in velocity becomes magnified if there are irregularities in the intimal surface. The insertion of a corrugated fabric graft into the arterial stream widens the zone of slow-moving blood at the periphery. The more slowly blood moves, the greater the propensity for clotting. Assuming that inflow pressure and distal resistance are constants, the velocity of blood flow in an interposed graft is inversely proportional to the square of the radius of the graft. Thus the velocity of blood flow in a 10-mm graft that runs into a 6-mm outflow vessel will be reduced to one-third of the velocity if a 6-mm graft had been used. This equation is visually perceptible when one attempts to use aortography to demonstrate lesions in the distal arterial tree in a patient with aortic and iliac aneurysmal disease. The flow velocity in the dilated arteries is so slow that accurate visualization of the distal arterial tree is often impossible. The slow flow in the aortic segment is the primary cause of the accumulation of mural thrombus in the even more slowly flowing blood in the periphery of the flow stream.

Another example of the clotting potential in a large inflow vessel that terminates in a small outflow system occurs when a common iliac artery or one limb of an aorta-femoral bifurcation graft becomes occluded. The maximum flow velocity is in the portion of the flow stream directed into the patent iliac outflow vessel. Distal aortic flow is reduced to a minimum except for the portion of its lumen supplying the outflow artery. As a consequence thrombus accumulates along the wall of the aorta proximal to the occluded iliac segment (**Fig. 2.39a–d**).

This illustration of blood flow dynamics has a pertinent clinical application when one selects the ideal procedure for thrombectomy of an occluded iliac limb of a bifurcation graft. Extraction of the thrombus by retrograde passage of a balloon catheter may fail to remove the loosely attached thrombus remaining on the aortic portion of the graft and set the stage for embolization into one or both of the iliac segments.

Fig. 2.39,a–d. Proximal progression of thrombus into aortic segment of bifurcation graft following occlusion of one of the iliac limbs. **a** pattern of blood flow at time of occlusion; **b** proximal propagation of thrombus.

c and d. Photographs of a portion of a resected 20 × 10-mm Dacron bifurcation graft which had been used as a bypass graft from the aorta to the common femoral arteries in a patient with aortoiliac and superficial femoral artery occlusive disease. The only outflow vessels were 6-mm profunda femoris arteries. The left iliac limb of the graft had been chronically occluded for several months and an attempt to reopen it by balloon thrombectomy was unsuccessful. The entire graft was removed and replaced by one of smaller size.

c The interior of the posterior half of the graft. Note the intact mural thrombus lining the right iliac limb of the graft. Thrombus in the left iliac limb has been removed by the balloon. The thick hemicircumferential layer of thrombus in the aortic portion has been fragmented during preparation of the specimen.

d A cross section of the graft cut from the top of the specimen before it was unroofed. The lumen, lined by fresh thrombus, is on the side of the patient iliac limb. The remainder of the graft is occupied by chronic thrombus on the side proximal to the occluded limb.

41

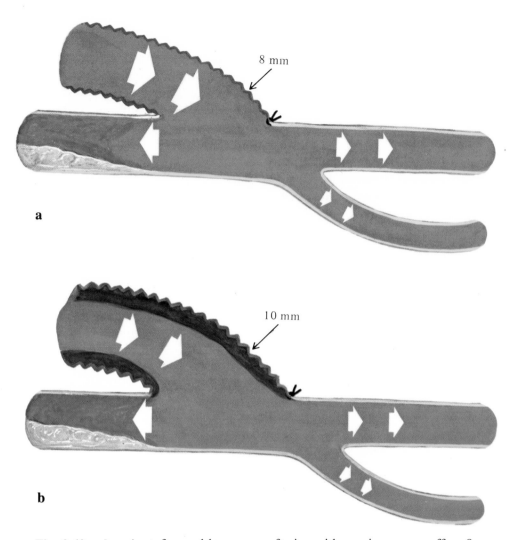

Fig. 2.40, a, b. Aortofemoral bypass; graft size with maximum run-off. **a** 8-mm iliac graft limb (maximum appropriate size for average adult male); **b** mural thrombus in 10-mm graft.

From the foregoing it follows that the most appropriate graft size is one that is comparable in size to the outflow vessel or vessels. **Fig. 2.40a** illustrates an appropriate 8-mm graft anastomosed to a common femoral artery in an adult male of average size when the outflow distally is into patent superficial femoral and profunda femoris arteries and proximally into the iliac artery. **Fig. 2.40b** illustrates a 10-mm graft in the same situation. The layer of thrombus that collects on the luminal surface of an oversize graft will usually be evident at a second operation (such as the repair of late false aneurysms) as a thin, gray layer of amorphous material which may be readily detached from the graft. It is probable that this laminated layer may be readily separated from the graft and fragmented with acute thigh flexion and thus become the cause of late graft occlusion. **Fig. 2.41 a and b** illustrates

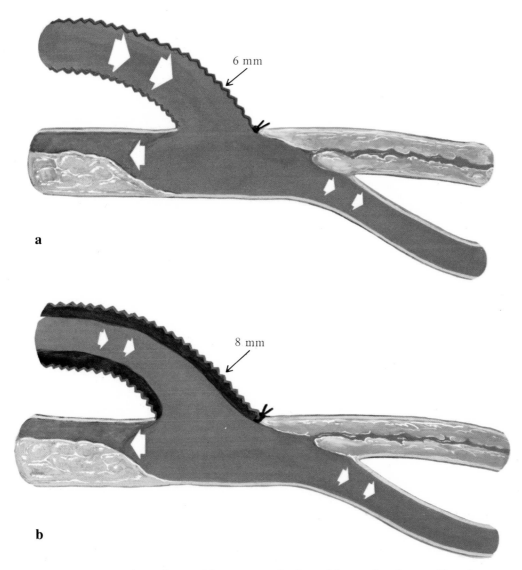

Fig. 2.41,a, b. Aortofemoral bypass; graft size with restricted run-off. **a** 6-mm iliac graft limb; **b** mural thrombus in an 8-mm graft.

comparable situations where 6- and 8-mm grafts are anastomosed to the common femoral artery when the profunda femoris is the only patent outflow artery, a vessel whose luminal diameter rarely exceeds 5 mm. The flow velocity in the larger graft will be approximately one-half of that in the smaller graft. **Fig. 2.42a–d** is a clinical result of the use of an oversize crossover graft in this situation.

The lesser gradient of laminar flow in a smooth-walled graft such as the saphenous vein may permit more tolerance in size disparity. Nevertheless, the gross disparity between the size of a normal saphenous vein anastomosed to a posterior tibial artery cannot be overlooked as a major factor in the high frequency of failure in femoral–tibial bypass grafting operations.

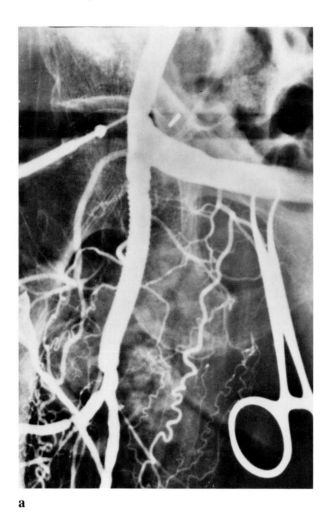

a

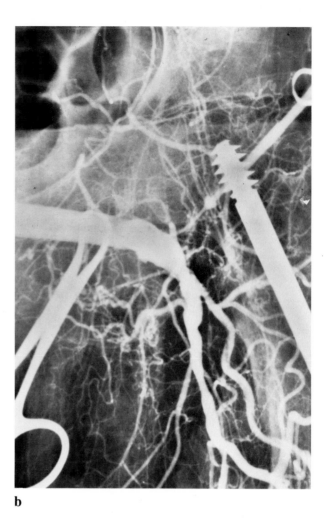

b

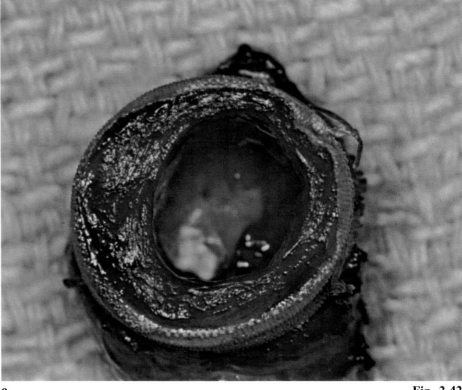

c

Fig. 2.42

44

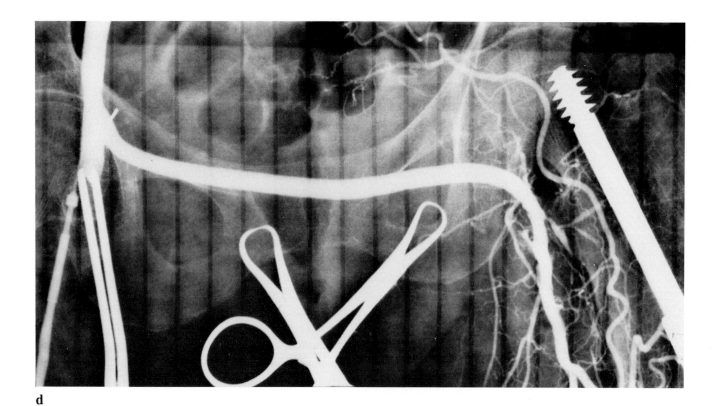

d

Fig. 2.42,a–d. Operative arteriograms showing the afferent (**a**) and efferent (**b**) ends of a 10-mm femoral crossover graft used in a patient with a previously placed aorta–bifemoral bypass graft in whom the left iliac arm of the graft had become occluded by atherosclerosis at the outflow site. Because of numerous previous abdominal operations, a crossover graft was used to revascularize the left profunda femoris artery.

One year later the patient returned with acute ischemia of the left leg secondary to thrombosis of the crossover graft. At operation, fresh thrombus was found in a graft that had become narrowed by a chronic circumferential thrombus reducing the lumen diameter to 5 mm, the size of the profunda femoris to which it had been attached. **c** End-on view of a cut section of the crossover graft. Most of the fresh thrombus has fallen from the lumen. The thick circumferential layer of old thrombus is a frequent finding when a graft larger than its outflow artery has been used. In this patient, the acute occlusion was presumably caused by disruption of the old thrombus caused by acute flexion of the thigh.

d A 6-mm graft was used to replace the previous 10-mm graft.

Extremity Skin Color During Operation

When a revascularization operation is performed on arteries within or supplying an extremity it becomes necessary to evaluate the adequacy of distal arterial perfusion as soon as possible after the occluding clamps are released. The absence of a normal pulse or the presence of a thrill in the arterial segment immediately distal to the reconstructed artery indicates, of course, a local problem in the operated segment that requires correction. The rapid return of a normal pulse at the ankle or the wrist, as the case may be, generally provides assurance that normal blood flow to the entire extremity has occurred. (The exception to this statement occurs in the patient who may have developed peripheral emboli to the small vessels in the foot or hand during the operation.)

The failure of the immediate appearance of peripheral pulses may be the result of one or more of three mechanisms: (1) preexisting distal occlusive disease; (2) intraoperative distal occlusion secondary to stasis thrombosis or embolization; or (3) vasoconstriction in the distal branches.

Temporary vasoconstriction in the arterial tree distal to the level of the proximal clamp occlusion during the operation is a phenomenon seen in its most extreme form after renal revascularization operations. A similar phenomenon may occur to a lesser degree in the peripheral arteries in the extremities following clamp occlusion of the iliac, femoral, or popliteal arteries (or comparable arteries in the upper extremities) for the time period usually required for a reconstructive arterial operation. Even when the distal arterial branches are free of obstructive pathology, the period of delay in return of palpable pedal pulses following lower extremity operations may vary from a few minutes to as long as 3–4 hours. The more lengthy periods for pulse return usually occur in patients who have become hypothermic during the operation. This is an inconstant phenomenon, as bounding pedal pulses may occur in some patients within a few seconds of clamp release.

When the failure of immediate pulse return is the result of intraoperative distal occlusion, early recognition of the cause is imperative since removal of the obstruction, if possible, should be performed before the operation is terminated.

The differentiation between vasoconstriction and acute distal arterial occlusion in the patient whose distal pulses do not appear at the final phase of operation can generally be made with reasonable accuracy by observa-

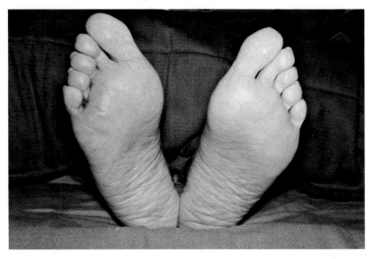

Fig. 2.43. View of soles of a patient's feet exposed for inspection during a lower extremity revascularization operation. Blood flow to the left foot has just been restored. Pinkness of the skin has progressively returned and has reached the base of the toes within 2 min indicating that no new obstructing lesion has appeared in the distal arterial tree during the operation. Blood flow to the right foot had been restored previously and the entire foot has regained its normal color.

tions of the rate and pattern of color return to the skin of the foot (usually the sole). Return of normal pink color begins first in the heel and progresses distally to the forefoot and toes (**Fig. 2.43**). In patients who have immediate return of pedal pulses, the color change begins within a few seconds of clamp release and involves the entire foot within 1–2 min. In the patient with vasoconstriction and an otherwise normal arterial tree, the first return of color may be delayed for 30–60 sec and progression to the toes is slow. An even more delayed return of color occurs in patients with preoperative chronic occlusion in arteries distal to the level of reconstruction. The presence of such lesions will usually have been determined in the preoperative evaluation. Whichever of these two mechanisms delay reperfusion, color is evenly distributed as it progresses up the foot. Although at first this color may be less than the brilliant pink of normal perfusion, the *progression* of color return signifies that a new occlusion has not occurred.

When distal occlusion has developed during the operation, the collateral channels that the patient with a preexisting chronic distal occlusion has developed will not be present. Pallor of the skin of the foot is profound, exceeds the customary pallor that occurs during the time of clamp occlusion, and persists for a lengthy period after release of the clamps. This alone indicates that remedial action must be taken. If color does return it will be deeply cyanotic and distributed unevenly in a mottled pattern on the sole of the foot.

Observation of color return is a necessary and routine observation, and in all patients undergoing arterial revascularization operations involving the extremities, the original draping is arranged to facilitate it. For aorta-iliac-common femoral operations the feet are left uncovered beneath the instrument table to permit inspection of the color of their soles and toes (**Fig. 2.44**). For more distal operations in the legs and for all operations in

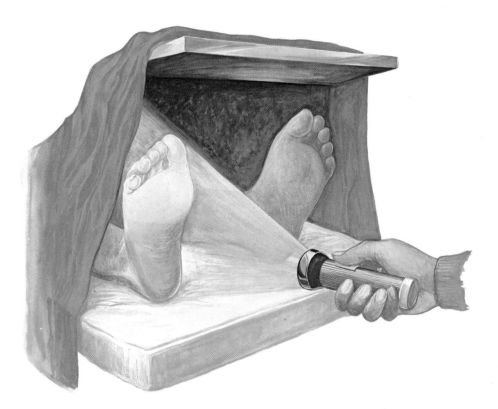

Fig. 2.44. Draping to leave feet exposed.

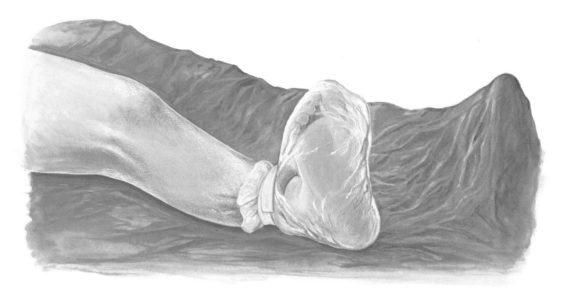

Fig. 2.45.   Leg draped free with plastic transparent covering on foot.

the upper extremities, the leg or arm is draped circumferentially using only a single layer of transparent plastic to cover the hand or foot (**Fig. 2.45**).

If any uncertainty exists as to the cause of poor foot color or lack of expected pedal or popliteal pulses, intraoperative arteriography is indicated. Usually this will clarify the problem and indicate the appropriate course of action. The routine use of Fogarty balloon catheters to overcome temporary vasoconstriction is not recommended. The phenomenon is reversible and does not warrant incurring intimal damage that the balloon occasionally creates.

Carotid Atherosclerosis

3

Carotid Bifurcation Endarterectomy

Of all the sites of atherosclerosis in the extracranial arteries supplying the brain, the region of the common carotid bifurcation is the most frequent and the most likely to be the cause of cerebral ischemia or infarction. The disease usually appears first in the short segment of normal bulbous enlargement of the first 2–4 cm of the internal carotid artery on the side opposite to the origin of the external carotid artery.

Progressive intimal thickening to the point of total arterial occlusion is a predictable event in most patients, provided they live long enough. This process may be accelerated by acute subintimal hemorrhage in the region of the carotid bulb. When occlusion occurs, the static column of blood in the undiseased distal internal carotid artery clots. The distal extent of thrombosis is determined by the volume of collateral blood flow from intracranial collaterals. If the volume is large, thrombus halts in the carotid siphon. If collaterals are inadequate, thrombosis extends distally into the middle cerebral artery resulting inevitably in cerebral infarction.

Thrombus in the carotid artery remains loosely attached to the arterial wall during the first 12–24 hours and can usually be extracted by grasping it with forceps through a proximal cervical carotid arteriotomy. Beyond this time period, a balloon catheter is needed to extract the clot if the catheter can be passed beyond the distal level of occlusion.

When the collateral blood supply to the ipsilateral hemisphere is sufficient to maintain adequate flow therein, carotid occlusion may produce transient symptoms or, more usually, no symptoms at all. Thus the only time that occlusion may come to attention clinically is when a neurologic deficit persists, usually as a result of cerebral infarction. If such is the case, early restoration of blood flow by endarterectomy and distal thrombectomy results in a greater morbidity as a result of intracranial hemorrhage than if the operation were not performed. A later operation in which a balloon catheter is used to extract the distal thrombus carries the prohibitive risk of creating an arteriovenous fistula in the carotid sinus. With the passage of time, the thrombus shrinks and organizes and the artery becomes no more than a fibrous cord (**Fig. 3.1**). Thus the demonstration of total occlusion of the internal carotid artery in a patient with a neurologic deficit becomes, in most instances, a contraindication to direct operation on the carotid artery.

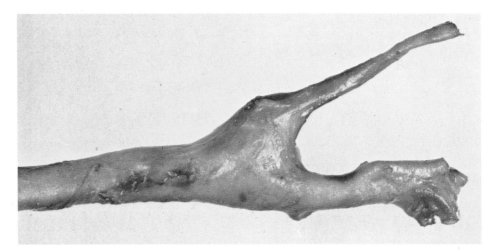

Fig. 3.1. Postmortem specimen of the carotid bifurcation in a patient who developed hemiplegia from atherosclerotic occlusion of the internal carotid artery 1 year before death. Note the shrunken cordlike internal carotid artery at the top.

As the original atheroma progresses, changes that in themselves may result in cerebral damage may occur before the development of total occlusion. Intramural hemorrhage within the carotid bulb may cause acute stenosis of the artery. Hemorrhage within the arterial wall may become the nidus for the accumulation of necrotic atheromatous debris, which may break into the lumen through an intimal ulcer and embolize to the brain. The craggy protuberance of the atheromatous intima into the lumen may create eddy currents conducive to mural thrombus, also a source of emboli. The friability of the various lesions in or adjacent to the arterial lumen may not be apparent on the preoperative arteriogram (**Figs. 3.2–3.11**).

Thus, exercising extreme care in mobilizing the diseased arterial segments becomes mandatory in all carotid operations for atherosclerosis. In the most common situation, the atheroma in the *internal* carotid artery terminates distally in a well-defined end point 1–3 cm beyond the end of the bulb, often ending as a sliver of thickened intima narrowed to a point. The distal intima is of normal thickness and retains its normal attachment to the underlying media. In less favorable situations, the gross atheroma comes to an end, but the distal intima retains a slightly greater than normal thickness and is easily separated from the underlying media, an abnormality that extends to the base of the skull. The end point in the external carotid artery is often poorly defined. Proximally, the full length of the common carotid intima is slightly thickened and freely detachable from the media.

Fig. 3.2,a, b. Endarterectomy specimen showing acute intramural hemorrhage into the wall of the internal carotid bulb. The patient had experienced an 8-hour episode of contralateral hemiparesis 3 days prior to arteriography and operation.

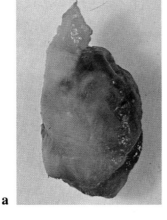

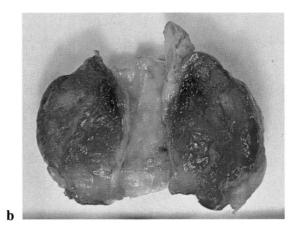

a

b

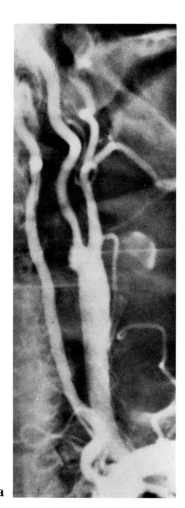

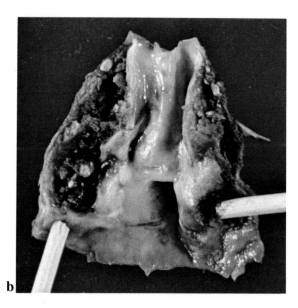

Fig. 3.3,a, b. Arteriogram (**a**) and endarterectomy specimen (**b**) in patient with recurrent hemispheric TIAs showing intramural accumulations of atherosclerotic debris and chronic hemorrhage. Intimal ulceration in the right lower corner had provided an opening for the release of microemboli.

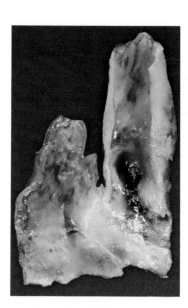

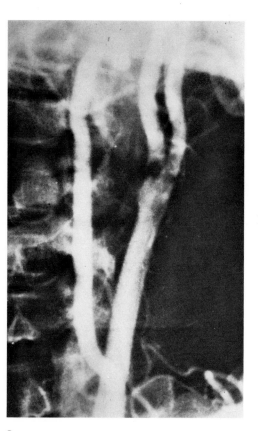

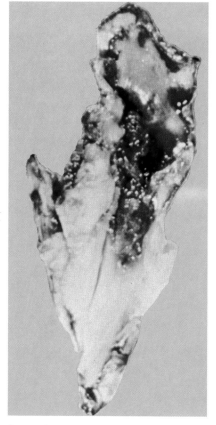

Fig. 3.4. Endarterectomy specimen showing a deep ulcer in the carotid bulb partially filled with fresh thrombus.

Fig. 3.5,a, b. Arteriogram (**a**) and endarterectomy specimen (**b**) showing advanced stenosis in the internal carotid segment and a loosely attached thrombus partially occluding the residual lumen.

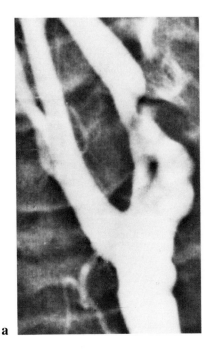

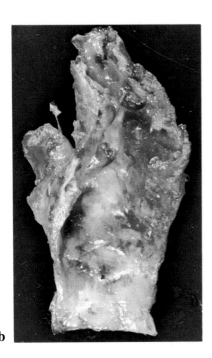

Fig. 3.6,a, b. Arteriogram (**a**) and endarterectomy specimen (**b**) showing gross atherosclerotic changes in terminal common carotid artery and the internal carotid bulb, as well as focal deposits of chronic mural thrombus.

a

b

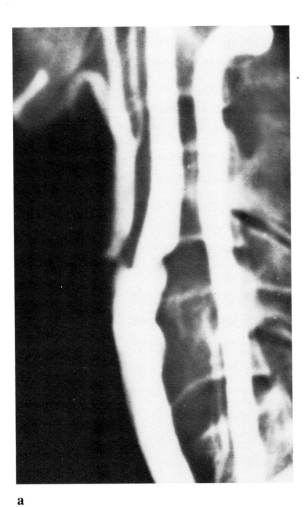

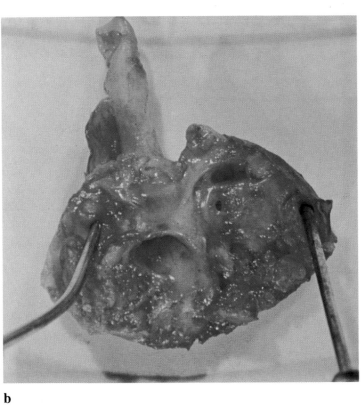

a

b

Fig. 3.7,a, b. Arteriogram (**a**) and endarterectomy specimen (**b**) showing extensive intimal degeneration in the full circumference of the common and internal carotid portions of the specimen.

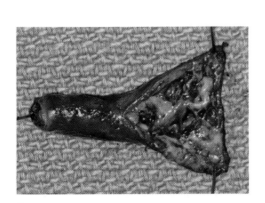
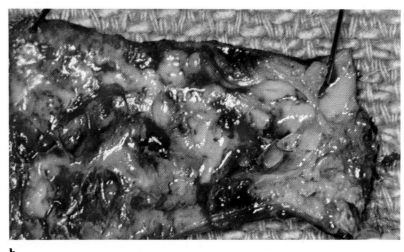

a   b

Fig. 3.8,a, b. Photographs of a resected distal common carotid artery in a patient with atherosclerosis confined to an area of extensive previous radiation for the treatment of pharyngeal malignancy. The artery has become shrunken and, in addition, almost occluded by the atheromatous lesions. The artery was replaced by an iliac artery autograft.

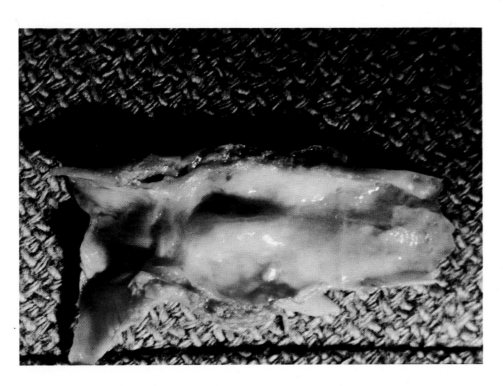

Fig. 3.9. Endarterectomy specimen with intramural deposits of granular degeneration exposed to the lumen through a small ulcer shown at the bottom of the specimen. Also shown is the tapered end point of the atherosclerotic lesion and a small fragment of grossly normal intima to the right.

53

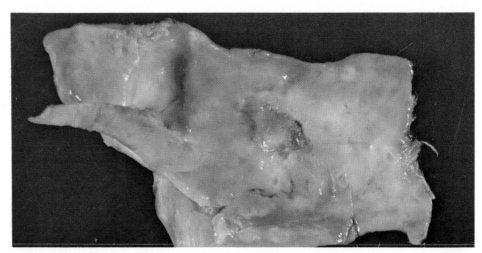

Fig. 3.10. Endarterectomy specimen showing an early stage of atherosclerosis in which an ulcer has already developed. The normal-appearing intima at the left end of the specimen is at the end point of disease in the distal internal carotid artery.

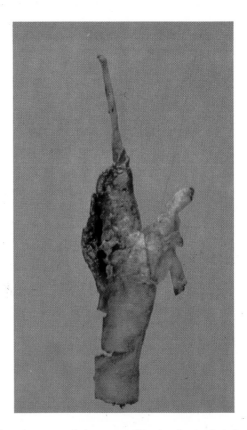

Fig. 3.11. Endarterectomy specimen showing mural degeneration in the bulb of the internal carotid and a long tongue of distal atheroma. Except for one other patient with unoperable disease extending to the bony foramen this is the longest distal extension of atherosclerosis we have encountered in over 2000 carotid endarterectomies.

All of the patients whose specimens are shown had had hemispheric TIAs. The fragility of most of the lesions is apparent. In many the arteriogram had failed to disclose an unstable lesion. These serve to emphasize the need for using particular care in the arterial mobilization portion of operation in all patients with suspected carotid atherosclerosis.

Technique

Approach and Preparation   The skin incision is made along the line of an existing skin crease and deepened through the platysma to the fibers of the sternocleidomastoid muscle (SCM) (**Fig. 3.12**). The incision is centered over the level of the common carotid bifurcation as determined by its distance from the horizontal ramus of the mandible demonstrated on the lateral projection of the selective preoperative carotid arteriogram. In any case, it should be at a level no closer than one fingerbreadth below the mandible in order to avoid severing the recurrent marginal mandibular branch of the facial nerve, which courses just beneath the platysma. A more vertical incision paralleling the common and internal carotid arteries leaves a permanent and unsightly scar. The scar of a skin-crease incision usually becomes hardly noticeable within 6 months of the operation.

The great auricular nerve, visible at the posterior end of the incision, should be preserved as its severance produces troublesome anesthesia of the ear and adjacent skin. If inadvertently severed, it should be reunited.

One or more of the anterior fibers of the cervical plexus will require division to facilitate the deeper development of the exposure. This division creates a zone of cutaneous anesthesia between the incision and the mandible that slowly lessens in area within the first year. The anterior jugular vein is also divided. The upper flap can then be developed by scalpel dis-

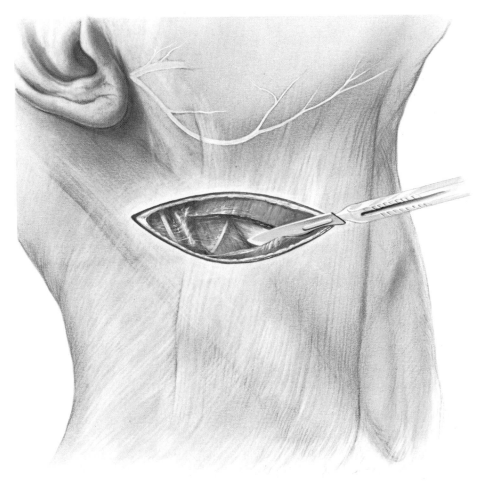

Fig. 3.12. Skin-crease incision.

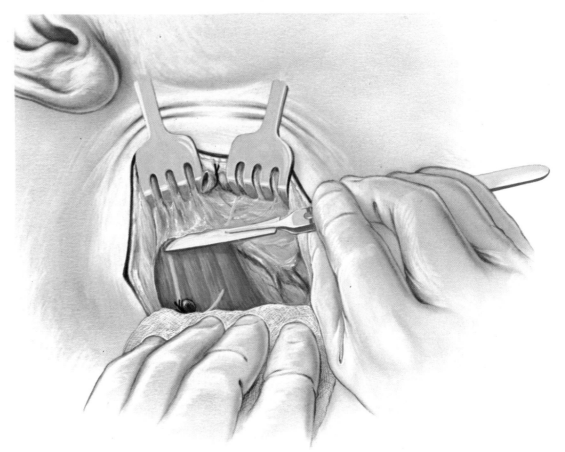

Fig. 3.13. Mobilization of upper flap.

section in a plane on the surface of the SCM (**Fig. 3.13**). Dissection at this level avoids the recurrent marginal mandibular branch of the facial nerve, which will be contained within the substance of the flap. Retraction injury to this nerve is rare and is evident by no more than a temporary inability to depress the ipsilateral corner of the lip.

The anterior edge and the adjacent posterior surface of the SCM are mobilized by scissor dissection (**Fig. 3.14**). Superiorly this portion of the dissection need go no further than the level of the mandible. Cephalad to this point the internal carotid artery is no longer under the cover of the SCM. Limiting the upper level of mobilization of the SCM at this point avoids damage to the spinal accessory nerve that enters the muscle at a higher level. The posterior reflection of the SCM is continued to the point where the internal jugular vein becomes visible. The lower flap is developed in the same plane (**Fig. 3.15**). The length of the arterial exposure is limited only by the length of the skin incision, which can be extended when necessary to produce a deeper flap.

A posterolateral approach to the carotid artery from the side of the jugular vein is the least vascular. A vertical incision in the sheath of the jugular vein extended superiorly as far as necessary will pass posterior to the hypoglossal nerve and prepares the field for a posterior approach to the carotid artery (**Fig. 3.16**). The carotid bifurcation is usually adjacent to the point of entry of the common facial vein.

The SCM and the jugular vein are retracted together after the vagus nerve has been identified. Inadvertent retraction of the vagus nerve often results in temporary or even permanent paresis of the fibers that become the recurrent laryngeal nerve. Vocal cord paresis is a recognized complica-

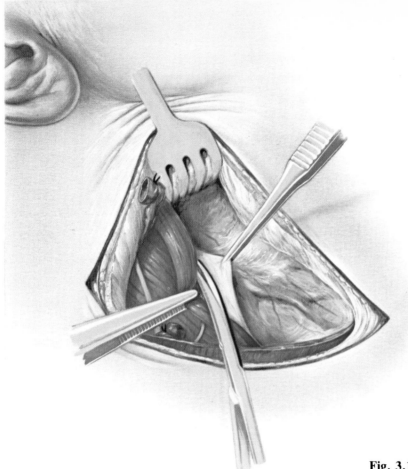

Fig. 3.14. Dissection of sternocleidomastoid muscle.

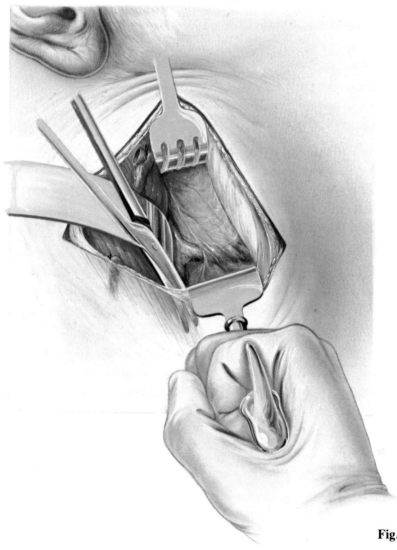

Fig. 3.15. Development of proximal dissection.

57

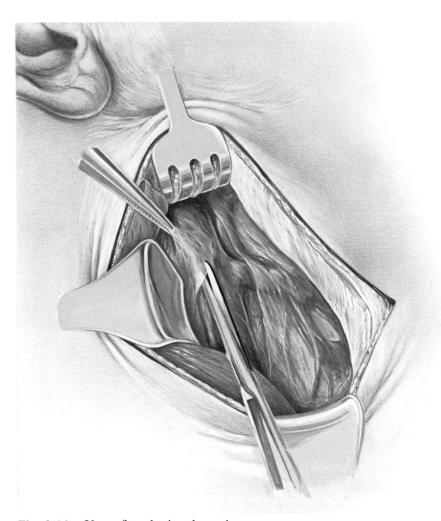

Fig. 3.16. Unroofing the jugular vein.

tion of carotid surgery and can largely be avoided by care in protection of the vagus nerve during this part of the dissection.

The carotid artery is approached midway between the parallel courses of the vagus nerve and the descendens hypoglossi nerve (**Fig. 3.17**). The latter supplies the muscles of deglutition and should be preserved whenever possible. Occasionally a twig of this nerve will connect with the vagus and require division to facilitate exposure. The vagus nerve occasionally occupies a position in the areolar tissue at the level of the carotid bulb more anterior than the one shown in the drawing. As the areolar incision is extended upward at the upper level of the carotid bulb, a small vascular bundle crossing the internal carotid artery between the external carotid artery and the SCM is encountered. The first portion of the hypoglossal nerve courses anterior and parallel to the distal internal carotid artery. It angles sharply forward after passing behind this bundle. Division of the artery and vein allows the hypoglossal nerve to assume a more anterior position and opens the space above for mobilization of the internal carotid artery to the upper level of the atherosclerotic lesion.

Rubber slings are passed to encircle the internal carotid artery *distal* to the bulb and the common carotid artery *proximal* to the lesion. Gentle traction on the slings allows the carotid bulb to be lifted for dissection of the areolar tissue from its posterior surface (**Fig. 3.18**). Direct traction on

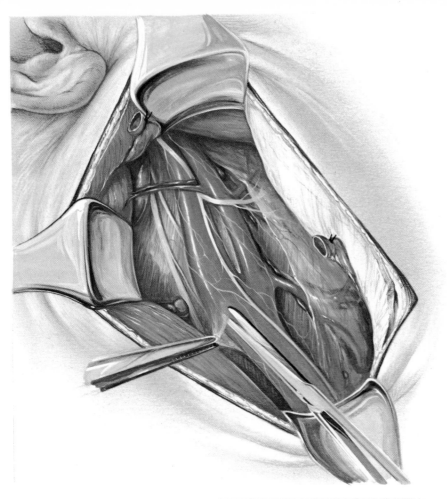

Fig. 3.17. Incision of carotid sheath.

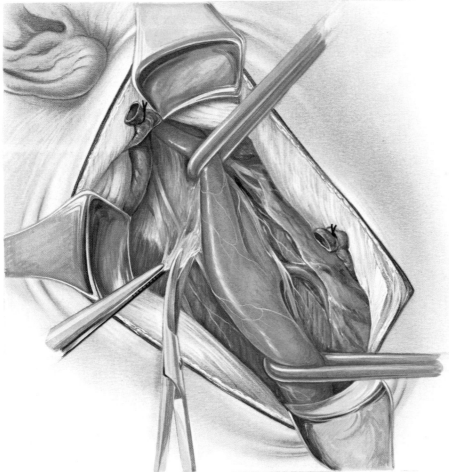

Fig. 3.18. Skeletonization of carotid artery.

59

the bulb or instrumental retraction of any portion of the bulb must be avoided in order to prevent dislodgment of clot or atherosclerotic debris within its lumen. The key phrase is to "dissect the patient away from the artery rather than the artery away from the patient." The dissection plane posteriorly should hug the artery in order to avoid damage to the superior laryngeal nerve, which crosses behind the bulb to reach its position adjacent to the superior laryngeal artery.

Digital palpation of the distal internal carotid artery over a curved clamp beyond the end of the bulb identifies the distal end of the atheroma, which customarily extends as a narrow tongue for 1–4 cm beyond the upper end of the bulb (**Fig. 3.19**).

Dissection of the areolar tissue from the anterior and posterior surfaces of the external carotid artery and its terminal branches clears the field for application of a specially designed clamp that occludes all of the terminal branches without the necessity of dissecting each one individually (**Figs. 3.20 and 3.21**).

Stump Pressure   The internal carotid stump pressure is obtained after clamp occlusion of the common and external carotid arteries. A 22-gauge needle connected by way of flexible tubing to a strain gauge and an oscilloscope is inserted into the common carotid artery proximal to the atherosclerotic lesion and distal to the common carotid clamp (**Fig. 3.21**). Since this arterial segment is a cul-de-sac, the presence of a stenotic lesion in the internal carotid artery distal to the needle does not influence the validity of the recorded pressure.

The stump pressure is an indicator of blood pressure within the ipsilateral cerebral hemisphere. This pressure can occur only as a result of collateral communications from the contralateral hemisphere and/or the vertebrobasilar system by way of the posterior communicating arteries. To the extent that blood pressure can be equated with blood flow, the stump pressure reflects the collateral flow in the hemisphere. Our own experience indicates that a stump pressure of 50 mm Hg or more demonstrates adequate hemispheric blood flow to maintain cellular function for a period of carotid occlusion in the time frame of a careful carotid endarterectomy (15–25 min). The noteworthy exception occurs in a patient with a prior occlu-

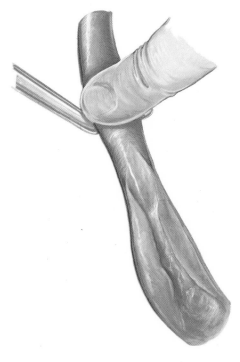

Fig. 3.19. Palpation to determine distal end point.

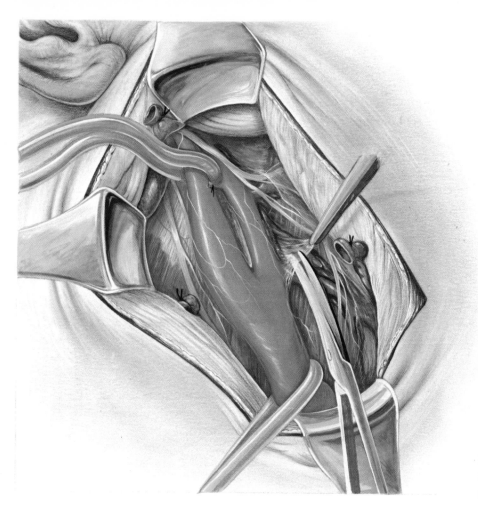

Fig. 3.20. Exposure of anterior surface of the external carotid artery.

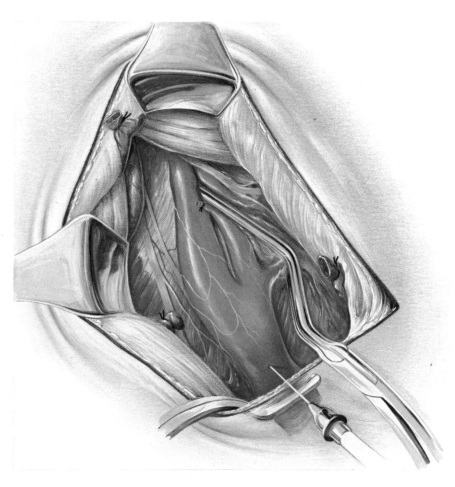

Fig. 3.21. Determination of stump pressure.

61

sion of the middle cerebral artery or one of its branches, in which circumstance the blood pressure in the arterial tree distal to the intracranial occlusion will be less than the internal carotid stump pressure. This becomes clinically relevant in patients with a previous infarct in the ipsilateral hemisphere for whom a stump pressure of 50 mm Hg may not reflect adequate collateral blood flow in the area adjacent to the previous infarct.

Patients with stump pressures in excess of 50 mm Hg, with the exception just noted, are operated upon without the use of an internal shunt. Stump pressure between 40 and 50 mm Hg may usually be elevated to more than 50 mm Hg by the induction of mild systemic hypertension. This technique becomes a useful alternative to using a shunt in the occasional patient with an abnormally high carotid bifurcation who, with a shunt in place, would present potential difficulties to exposure of the atherosclerotic end point. Elevation of the systemic systolic blood pressure by vasoconstrictive drugs to levels in excess of 180 mm Hg introduces the risk of myocardial ischemia and should be avoided.

An intraoperative decrease of the systemic blood pressure will decrease the stump pressure proportionately. If the measured stump pressure was in the range of 50 mm Hg, a subsequent fall in systemic pressure, should it occur during the period of carotid occlusion, will result in inadequate blood flow to the ipsilateral hemisphere. Continuous recording of the systemic blood pressure by a radial artery pressure line during the course of any carotid operation is thus highly desirable.

For surgeons who customarily perform endarterectomy in the presence of a shunt in all patients, the issues just discussed are of only passing interest. In our own experience the presence of a shunt magnifies the occasional difficulty in creating an adequate end point. The demonstration of a high stump pressure allows for the performance of a careful, unhurried operation with unimpeded access for performing the critical maneuvers in the distal internal carotid artery.

Endarterectomy Bradycardia and hypotension may appear during dissection in the region of the carotid sinus. Two milliliters of 2% lidocaine injected into this area produces a prompt return of normal blood pressure and heart rate.

Prior to the final application of the occluding clamps, systemic heparinization is instituted primarily to prevent clotting in the static column of blood in the distal cervical internal carotid artery. For 25 min of occlusion, 2500–3500 units is adequate for this purpose.

The clamps used for the common carotid and internal carotid have been designed with an extra curve to permit occlusion of the arteries at more proximal and distal levels than can be accomplished with conventional clamps. The clamps are applied laterally and then rotated anteriorly to expose the surface of the diseased arterial segment between them (**Fig. 3.22a and b**). A longitudinal arteriotomy is made in the wall of the common and internal carotid arteries directly opposite the orifice of the external carotid artery (**Fig. 3.23**). If the artery is not rotated, the incision will lie adjacent to the external carotid artery often making alignment for its subsequent closure inaccurate. Unless there is a palpable lesion extending for a lengthy distance into the internal carotid artery, the arteriotomy is terminated immediately proximal to the distal end of the carotid bulb. If a satisfactory end point for the endarterectomy can be developed through this incision, the arteriotomy can be closed without concern for narrowing of the outflow vessel.

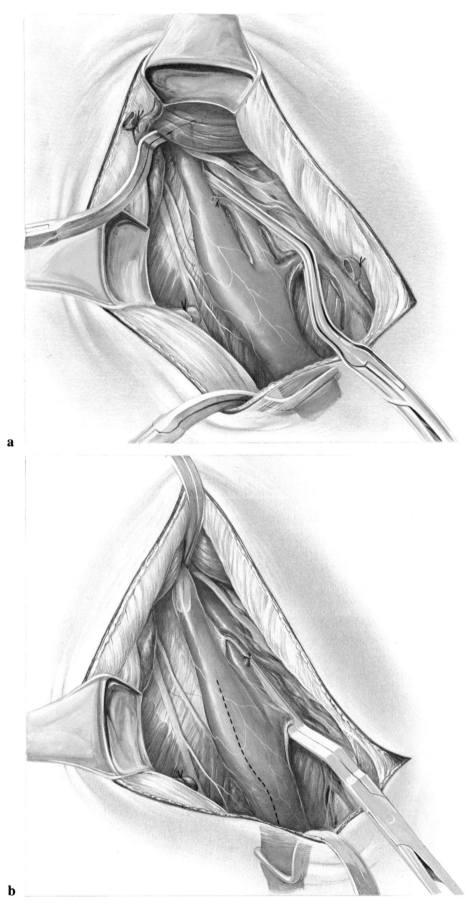

a

b

Fig. 3.22,a, b. Preparation for arteriotomy. **a** common and internal clamps applied laterally; **b** clamps rotated anteriorly.

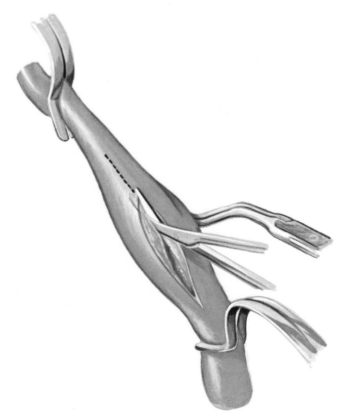

Fig. 3.23. Position of arteriotomy.

The endarterectomy dissection plane is developed first at the level of maximum disease. As with endarterectomy elsewhere, the correct plane is easily recognized. The medial surface that remains is smooth and has a color hue similar to that of muscle. The specimen side of the plane is also smooth and has the creamy yellow hue of an atheroma. Once the plane has been developed to the depth of the artery, a special sharply curved clamp is used to continue the dissection to the opposite side of the arteriotomy (**Fig. 3.24a and b**). The intima in the unopened artery between the proximal occluding clamp and the end of the arteriotomy is easily separable from the media by the insertion and spreading of the jaws of an angled hemostat (**Fig. 3.25**). The intimal core must be transected cleanly to avoid the creation of loose tags that may break free or become the nidus for a mural thrombus. Introducing the curved blades of dissecting scissors beneath the edges of the arteriotomy will accomplish a clean transection (**Fig. 3.26**).

An alternate and generally preferable method is to crush the artery immediately distal to the proximal clamp with a hemostat, fracturing the intima cleanly without apparent damage to the outer layers of the artery. Cephalad traction on the specimen withdraws a cylinder of atheromatous intima with a clean end point (**Fig. 3.27a and b**).

The intimal core in the orifice of the external carotid artery is removed by eversion endarterectomy, pushing the media away from the central core of atherosclerotic intima (**Fig. 3.28a**). A tongue of thickened intima occasionally extends beyond the location of the occluding clamp. Momentary release of this clamp (with a suction in place) allows the specimen to be extracted with gentle instrumentation (**Fig. 3.28b**). Failure to remove all of the thickened external carotid intima may be of no real consequence to the patient, provided the internal carotid is patent, but residual stenosis may

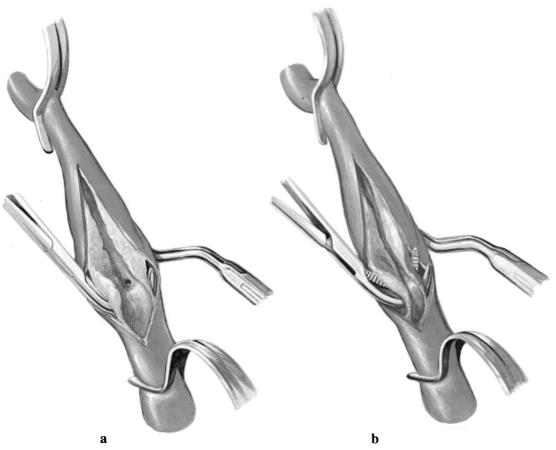

a   b

Fig. 3.24,a, b. Development of endarterectomy plane. **a** separation at point of maximum disease; **b** extension around the circumference.

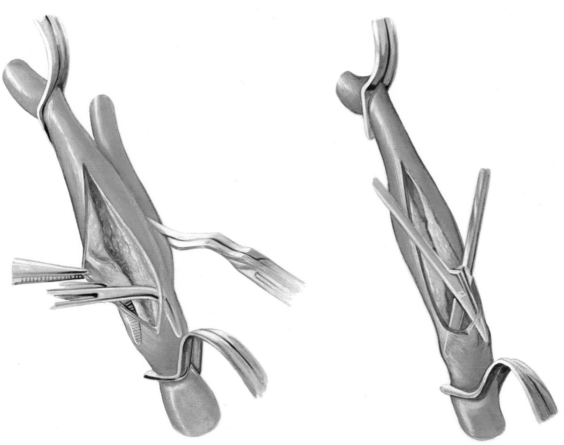

Fig. 3.25. Proximal dissection.   **Fig. 3.26.** Transection of proximal intimal core.

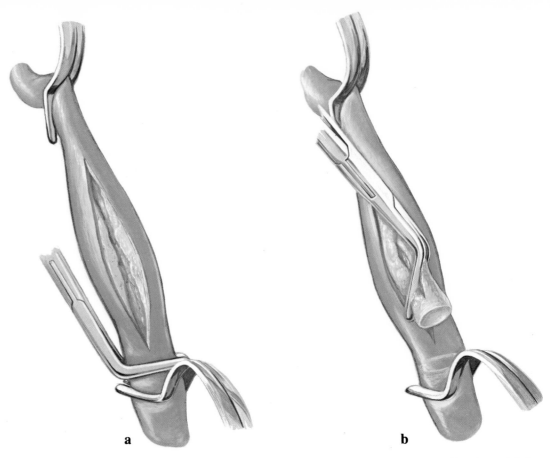

Fig. 3.27,a, b. Crushing technique for proximal end point. **a** application of right-angle clamp; **b** extraction of proximal core.

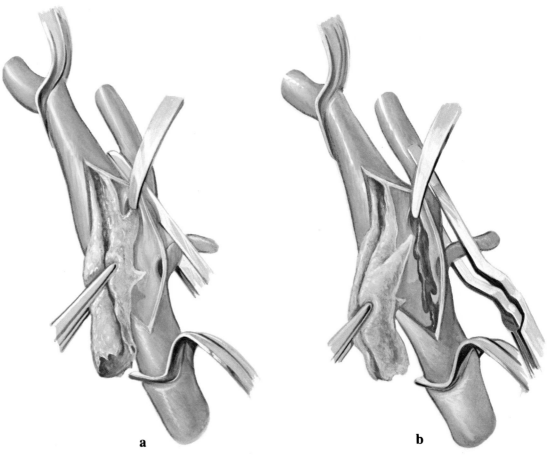

Fig. 3.28,a, b. Removal of external carotid portion of lesion. **a** endarterectomy to level of clamp; **b** distal extraction with clamp released momentarily.

66

produce a bruit that may confuse evaluation on subsequent follow-up examination.

A more precise external carotid endarterectomy is required in patients in whom the internal carotid artery is occluded and stenosis of the external carotid artery reduces the effectiveness of this artery as a source of collateral blood flow to the ipsilateral cerebral hemisphere. In this situation, it is preferable to open the external carotid artery with a longitudinal arteriotomy, develop a satisfactory end point, and close the arteriotomy with a vein patch. In view of the recent introduction of bypass grafts from the superficial temporal artery to an intracranial artery in patients with occlusion of the internal carotid artery, the creation of an unimpeded inflow channel in the external carotid artery has become particularly important.

The development of the end point in the internal carotid artery is the critical portion of the operation. When the atheroma extends beyond the arteriotomy, its removal is facilitated if an assistant brings the common and internal artery clamps closer to one another, permitting a partial eversion endarterectomy as the dissector pushes the media away from the specimen (**Fig. 3.29**). The specimen usually separates cleanly at the junction of diseased and normal intima. The specimen that shows a thin, feathered and tapered tip provides assurance that a complete endarterectomy has been performed.

In most cases the distal end point will be a sharply defined line of demarcation. Residual intimal tags at the end point or proximal to it should be carefully teased free by circumferential traction (**Fig. 3.30a and b**). At this stage of the procedure the endarterectomized layer may tend to fall sharply downward from the distal intact internal carotid artery, giving the illusion of a residual ledge. Reduction of the eversion by distraction of the occluding clamps permits visual and instrumental appraisal of the adequacy of the

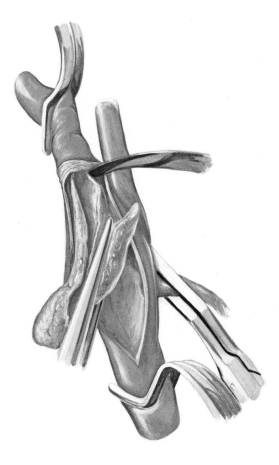

Fig. 3.29. Eversion endarterectomy of distal internal carotid lesion beyond end of the arteriotomy.

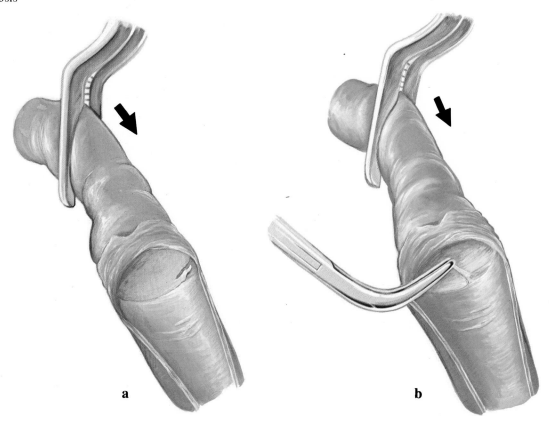

Fig. 3.30,a, b. Management of end point. **a** residual intimal tag; **b** circumferential extraction of tag.

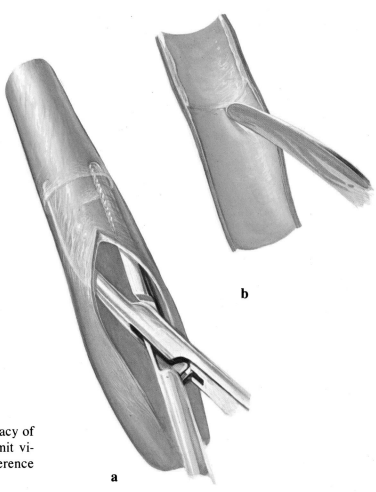

Fig. 3.31,a, b. Determination of adequacy of end point. **a** insertion of clamp to permit visual inspection; **b** testing intimal adherence with tip of dissector.

end point. With the edges of the arteriotomy held apart and the apex lifted with a blunt hook, the firmness of the attachment of the distal intima can be tested with the tip of the dissector (**Fig. 3.31a and b**).

In some types of atherosclerosis, normal-appearing intima distal to the end of the atheroma will be so loosely attached to the media that a secure end point cannot be reached. Nothing will be gained by attempting to continue the dissection distally since this abnormality continues to the base of the skull. If, when tested with the tip of the dissector, intimal adherence is less than normal the arteriotomy should be extended beyond the end point (**Fig. 3.32a and b**). Double-ended 7–0 tack-down sutures tied externally prevent a subsequent intramural dissection (**Fig. 3.33a and b**).

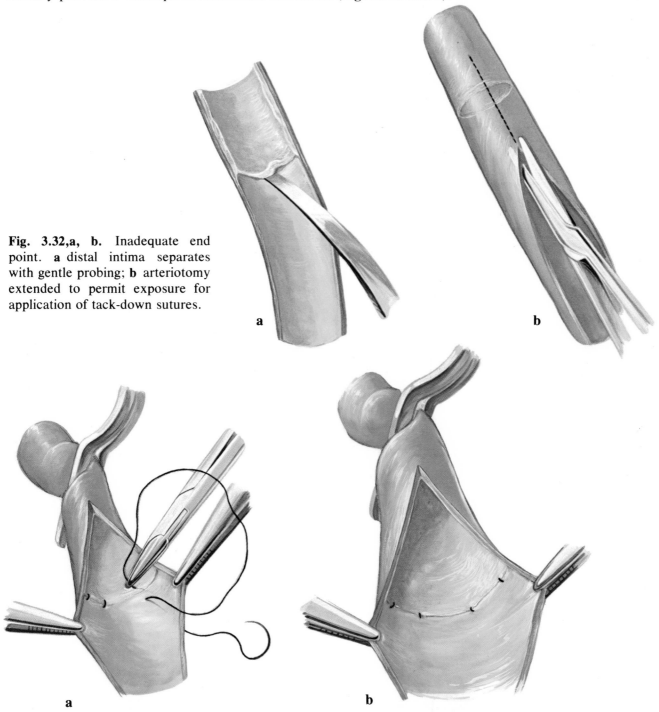

Fig. 3.32,a, b. Inadequate end point. **a** distal intima separates with gentle probing; **b** arteriotomy extended to permit exposure for application of tack-down sutures.

a

b

a

b

Fig. 3.33,a, b. Suture of distal intima. **a** insertion of tack-down sutures; **b** intima secured.

Closure The arteriotomy is closed with a continuous 6–0 suture. If the sutures beyond the end of the bulb are placed 1 mm deep and 1 mm apart, the postclosure narrowing of the artery will be barely perceptible. Once the suture line reaches the bulb, the sutures may be widened and deepened without concern for narrowing the bulb to less than the dimensions of the distal artery (**Fig. 3.34a and b**).

Careful attention to the fine details of closure of the arteriotomy should restore a normal contour to the carotid bulb and the distal internal carotid artery and avoid the need for widening the artery with a supplementary patch. Application of a patch merely adds another suture line upon which platelets or thrombus may accumulate or produces an aneurysmal bulge in the arterial lumen vulnerable to the later development of a mural thrombus.

Before placing the final sutures, the three clamps are individually and momentarily released to flush away residual fragments and trapped air. The internal carotid clamp is moved to a more proximal level to close the cul-de-sac into which intimal fragments could enter with final release of the clamps (**Fig. 3.35**). After closure of the arteriotomy, the external carotid is the first artery opened to forward flow to permit a final opportunity for flushing into a safe area. The clamp on the common carotid artery is released next and, finally, the internal carotid clamp.

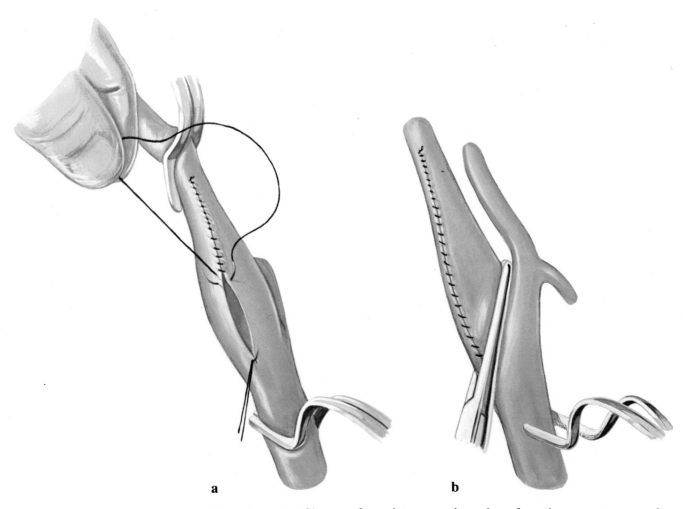

a   b

Fig. 3.34,a, b. Closure of arteriotomy. **a** insertion of continuous suture starting at distal end; **b** flow restored first into external carotid after repositioning of internal carotid clamp.

After release of all clamps, the endarterectomized arterial segment is carefully inspected and palpated. Although a rare occurrence, a palpable ledge or a thrill at the distal end point indicates the need for revision at that site. A sharp zone of stenosis may result from incorporating excessive adventitial fibers in the suture line. The constriction may be corrected by dissecting away the strands of adventitia adjacent to the suture line.

Stenosis may also occur from malalignment of the arteriotomy closure. This, of course, should not occur if a straight arteriotomy has been made. When the arterial wall is densely calcified, the blades of the scissors may be deflected, resulting in a zig-zag opening. If substantial stenosis occurs (or if the wall of the bulb has been damaged during the endarterectomy), a simple solution is to close the carotid bulb and anastomose the external carotid artery to the distal internal carotid artery (**Figs. 3.35 and 3.36a and b**).

Internal Shunt For reasons cited previously, an internal shunt will be required in approximately 20% of carotid bifurcation operations. We have found the Javid shunt with its special clamps to be admirably designed to create the least degree of intimal trauma. The tubing is only slightly smaller than the artery, and the concave blades of the clamps avoid the intimal disruption that a tourniquet occlusion tends to produce.

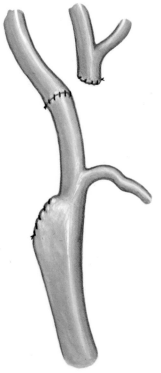

Fig. 3.35. External carotid–internal carotid anastomosis.

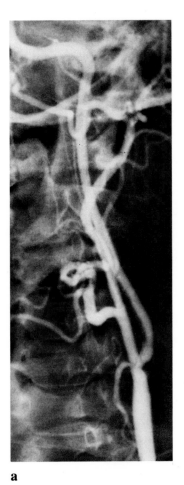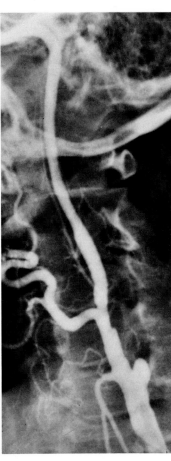

a   b

Fig. 3.36,a, b. Arteriograms (**a** preoperative; **b** postoperative) in a patient who had an external carotid–internal carotid transposition operation. Disruption of the carotid bulb had developed when a conventional endarterectomy was attempted.

71

The arteriotomy should be extended at both ends to a point beyond the end of visible disease (**Fig. 3.37**). A shorter incision risks separation of the intima when the shunt is inserted. The smaller end of the shunt is inserted into the distal internal carotid artery. When its position is secure, the distal clamp is released and the shunt advanced to a level several centimeters distal to the arteriotomy (**Fig. 3.38**).

The internal carotid Javid clamp is applied and the shunt withdrawn until the olive bulge of the shunt engages the clamp. After backbleeding fills the shunt with blood, the shunt is temporarily occluded with a hemostat (**Fig. 3.39**).

The proximal end of the shunt is then positioned for insertion into the common carotid artery. The cul-de-sac in the artery is filled with blood to displace any air bubbles releasing the clamp on the shunt. At this point, it is desirable to replace the proximal occluding clamp with thumb and finger compression as the proximal end of the shunt is advanced into position (**Fig. 3.40**). This is most easily accomplished by insertion of the index finger behind the artery below the lower flap and positioning the thumb externally on the surface of the neck. The beginning of the endarterectomy with blood flowing through the shunt is shown in **Fig. 3.41**. The ischemia time for insertion of the shunt is usually less than 2–3 min, a period within the limits of cerebral tolerance. **Fig. 3.42a and b** is an operative photograph of a Javid shunt in position.

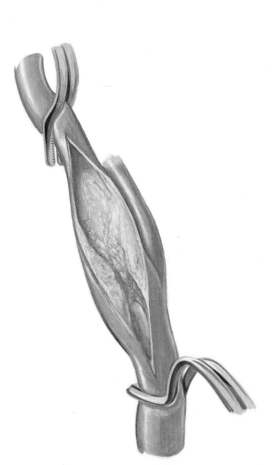

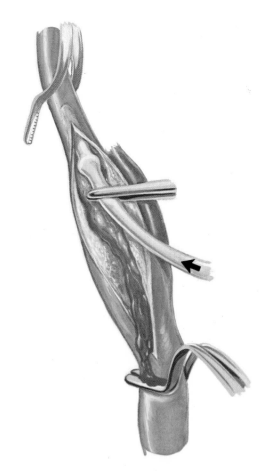

Fig. 3.37. Extended arteriotomy in preparation for shunt insertion.

Fig. 3.38. Insertion of distal end of shunt.

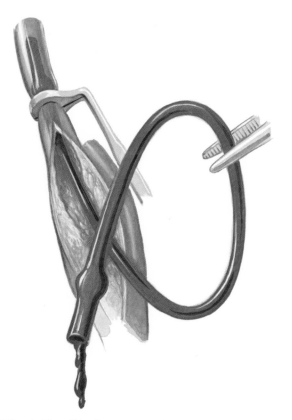

Fig. 3.39. Displacement of air from shunt.

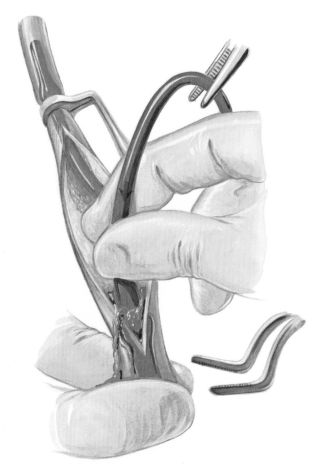

Fig. 3.40. Displacement of air from the common carotid artery.

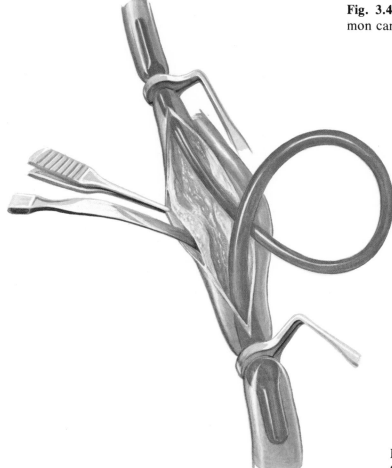

Fig. 3.41. Endarterectomy with functioning shunt in place.

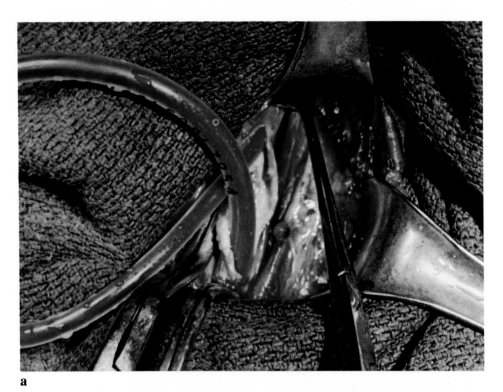

a

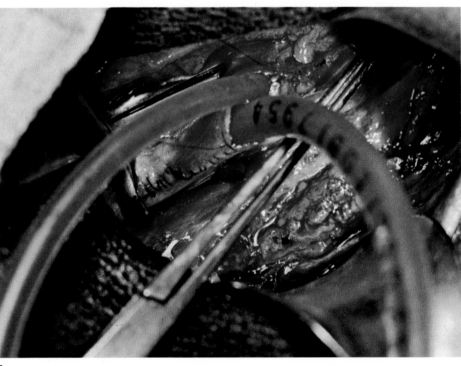

b

Fig. 3.42,a, b. Operative photographs of a Javid shunt in place in a patient with a carotid stump pressure less than 50 mm Hg. **a** The arteriotomy has been extended well beyond the end of visible disease. The external diameter of the distal end of the shunt is nearly that of the internal diameter of the internal carotid artery, which allows the Javid clamp (top) to be placed with minimal disruption of the intima. **b** The arteriotomy has been closed from each end to the point of emergence of the shunt.

Following completion of the endarterectomy, the arteriotomy is closed from each end to the point of exit of the shunt tubing (**Fig. 3.43**). The shunt is removed in the reverse order of its insertion. A partially occluding clamp is applied to allow restoration of blood flow during placement of the final sutures (**Fig. 3.44a and b**).

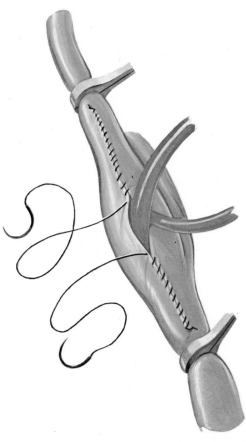

Fig. 3.43. Partial closure of arteriotomy with shunt in place.

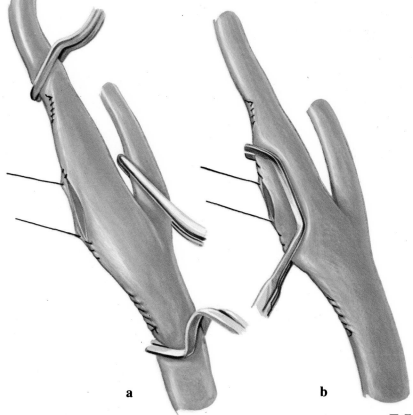

Fig. 3.44,a, b. Completion of closure. **a** shunt removed and clamps reapplied; **b** application of partially occluding clamp to restore blood flow.

a

b

75

Recurrent Carotid Stenosis

Recurrence of carotid stenosis at the site of a previous endarterectomy is a rare but recognized late sequela of endarterectomy at the carotid bifurcation and may develop in 1%–3% of patients as a result of one of two apparently separate pathologic processes. One is a new atherosclerotic lesion. In our series, the average time for the reappearance of atherosclerotic stenosis is 5–6 years. None has developed before the end of the second year. Stenosis may also develop from an unusual fibroplastic reaction on the surface of the endarterectomized arterial wall. This typically occurs within the first year after operation.

A residual bruit is often present after a satisfactory endarterectomy. Most commonly it is due to an inadequate endarterectomy end point of the poorly visualized external carotid atheroma. Thus the diagnosis of recurrent stenosis is usually made by a change in the quality of the bruit or by the development of new localizing symptoms of cerebral insufficiency.

The surgical technique for correcting the stenosis is basically the same as that for the primary lesion. If the lesion is atherosclerotic, a new endarterectomy plane can be developed without difficulty. If the lesion is fibroplastic, the new tissue can be removed only by sharp dissection with a scalpel.

The development of either type of lesion suggests that the patient is susceptible to further problems. This is the one situation for which patch graft closure of the arteriotomy is indicated. An elliptical segment of saphenous vein (taken from the ankle) is used to produce a deliberately oversized lumen for the purpose of delaying the hemodynamic effect if stenosis is to occur again. The carotid arteriograms and operative photographs of a patient with recurrent carotid stenosis caused by intimal fibroplasia are shown in **Fig. 3.45a–f.**

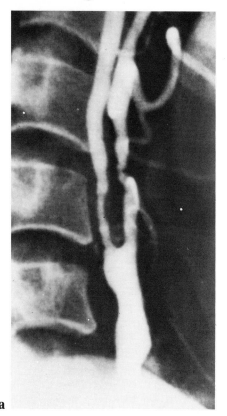 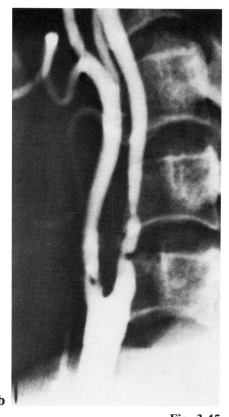

a b

Fig. 3.45

76

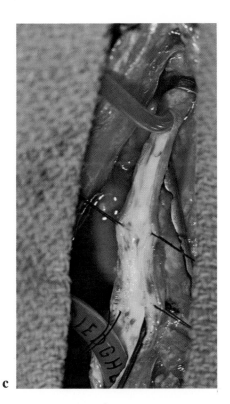

c

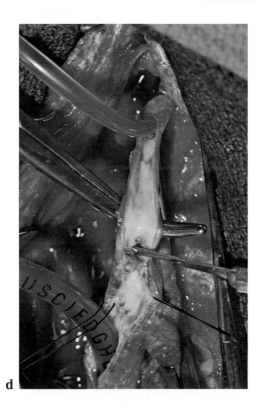

d

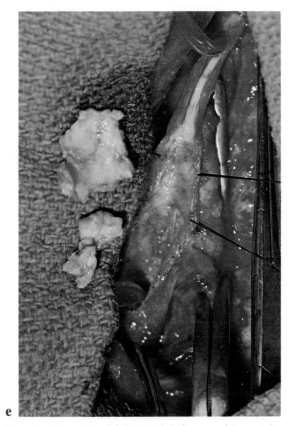

e

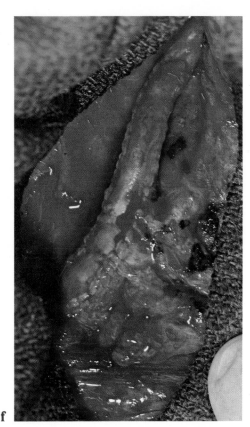

f

Fig. 3.45. **a, b** Right and left carotid arteriograms and operative photographs of a patient with bilateral recurrent carotid stenosis appearing within one year of carotid endarterectomy. Note the pale, thick, glistening mass of new tissue within the lumen (c).

c, d A scalpel with a Beaver blade is used to trim away the layer of rubbery fibrous tissue (d, e).

e, f The closure is augmented with a gusset of saphenous vein to prevent or postpone the effects of further fibrous overgrowth (f). [From Stoney and String: Recurrent carotid stenosis. Surgery, 80(6):705–710, December 1976 (Fig. 3).]

Common Carotid Endarterectomy

Atherosclerotic occlusion of the common carotid artery usually occurs as a result of disease at the carotid bifurcation that has advanced to total occlusion at this level. A much rarer site of the primary lesion is the left common carotid orifice on the aortic arch. We have never encountered a patient in whom the primary lesion of the right common carotid artery was at its proximal orifice. Primary lesions in the middle third of either artery are also rare except in patients who have had previous irradiation to the neck. An unusual case in which internal carotid atherosclerosis is associated with extensive disease in the common carotid artery is illustrated in **Fig. 3.46a–c.**

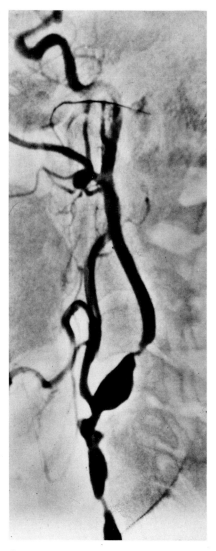

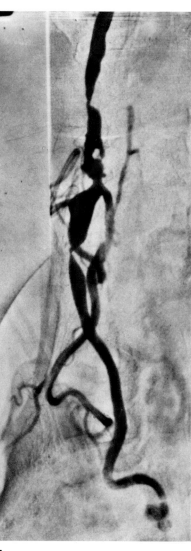

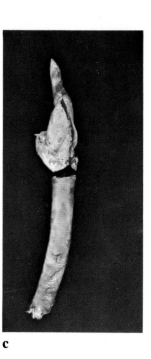

c

a   b

Fig. 3.46,a–c. Arteriograms of the left carotid artery in the anterior (**a**) and lateral (**b**) projections showing the unusual finding of advanced atherosclerosis in the common carotid artery as well as in the internal carotid bulb. A conventional open bifurcation endarterectomy was followed by closed endarterectomy of the distal two-thirds of the common carotid artery using the arterial stripper. **c** Photograph of the operative specimen.

When the original occlusion develops in the distal portion of the common carotid artery itself, patency of the internal and external carotid artery may be maintained even though some degree of atherosclerosis will be present in their proximal portions. In this circumstance, collateral blood flow to the ipsilateral hemisphere is supplied in part through arterial connections across the head and neck from the branches of the contralateral external carotid artery (Fig. 3.47a).

When retrograde thrombosis of the common carotid artery occurs as a result of occlusion of both the internal and external carotid arteries, thrombus in the internal carotid propagates to the intracranial position of the major carotid branches where collateral blood flow reenters the system. Occlusion of the external carotid artery, however, remains confined to its first few centimeters (Fig. 3.47b).

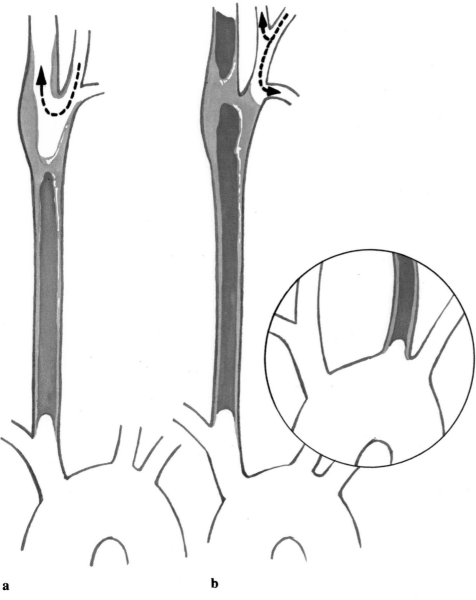

a b

Fig. 3.47, a, b. Patterns of common carotid occlusion. a primary occluding lesion confined to distal common carotid artery; b primary lesion involving the internal and external carotid orifices; inset proximal extension of thrombus when left common carotid becomes occluded.

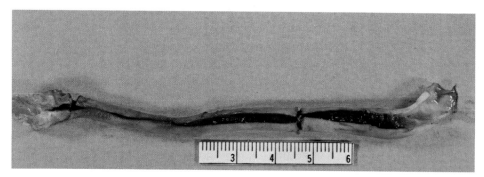

Fig. 3.48. Endarterectomy specimen in a patient with atherosclerotic occlusion of the right common carotid artery. Thrombosis occurred as the result of progression to occlusion of an atheroma at the common carotid bifurcation (top). Thrombus then developed in the static column of blood proximal to it. Note that the first 1–2 cm of the common carotid artery has remained patent. This is an almost constant finding and allows for safe application of an arterial clamp onto the proximal common carotid artery through a cervical approach. The specimen has been removed by open endarterectomy at the bifurcation and the retrograde passage of an arterial stripper.

Whatever the level of the original distal lesion, the static column of blood proximal to the occlusion clots. Thrombosis propagates retrograde to within 1–3 cm of the common carotid origin, i.e., the innominate bifurcation on the right and the aorta on the left (**Fig. 3.48**). Although gross atherosclerosis is only rarely encountered in the proximal two-thirds of the common carotid arteries, the normal adherence between the intima and media is absent and endarterectomy can be accomplished with ease in the usual subintimal dissection plane.

Many patients with either of the types of lesions shown in Fig. 3.47a and b will have escaped the development of frank stroke. Symptoms, when present, are those of chronic or transient decrease in cerebral or ocular perfusion, which may be sufficiently disabling to indicate operation. Patients with the lesion shown in Fig. 3.47a often have substantial atherosclerosis in the still-patent bulb of the internal carotid artery. If progression of the disease at this point results in internal carotid occlusion, the patient is at greater risk of stroke than if the external carotid artery were to be furnishing its normal collateral contribution to the cerebral hemisphere from a patent common carotid artery. For this reason the radiologic demonstration of common carotid occlusion even in the absence of symptoms indicates operation in patients who have retained patency of the internal carotid artery (Fig. 3.47a).

For patients with the more extensive lesion shown in Fig. 3.47b, operation to restore forward flow into the external carotid artery is indicated only if ipsilateral symptoms of reduced cerebral or retinal perfusion are present. In this case the objective of the operation is to increase collateral blood flow between the external carotid and the ophthalmic arteries or to provide normal forward flow into the superficial temporal artery in preparation for a temporal artery–intracranial bypass operation.

The ease of dissection in the wall of the common carotid artery in the customary endarterectomy plane has been a constant finding, and for this reason endarterectomy is the operation of choice for common carotid artery thrombosis. Full-length endarterectomy is the definitive procedure for occlusion on the right, since both ends of the occluded segment are accessible through cervical incisions.

Operative access to the common carotid artery is obtained through the conventional skin crease incision at the carotid bifurcation and a second transverse incision above the clavicle. The arterial segment between the incisions is mobilized by instrumental and finger dissection (**Fig. 3.49**). The distal atherosclerotic lesion in the carotid bifurcation is removed in the customary manner. On the right side, the proximal arterial clamp is placed across the common carotid artery just distal to the subclavian artery and proximal to the end of the thrombus. The proximal end point of the endarterectomy is usually simple to create by crushing the artery with an angled hemostat (**Fig. 3.50a**). A stripper of appropriate size is then introduced to surround the distal intimal core. The stripper can be passed with minimal resistance to the level of the proximal clamp (**Fig. 3.50b**). Since the intima at this level has been essentially transected by the crushing hemostat, the entire specimen may be withdrawn from the distal arteriotomy (**Fig. 3.50c**). In the rare circumstance in which the maneuver described above fails to transect the proximal intima, dividing it through a proximal arteriotomy may become necessary (**Fig. 3.51**).

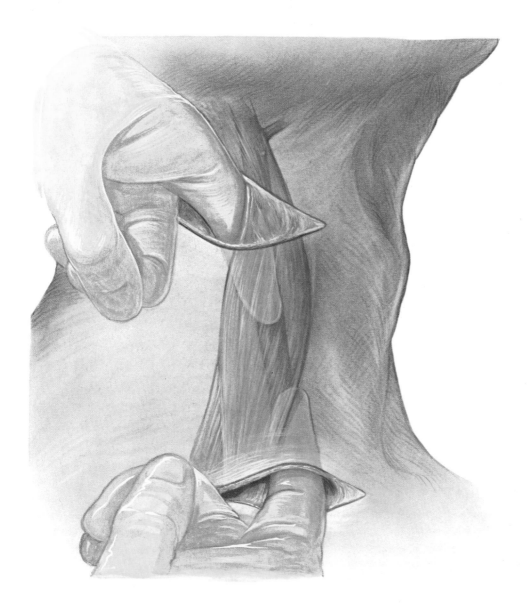

Fig. 3.49. Mobilization of right common carotid artery.

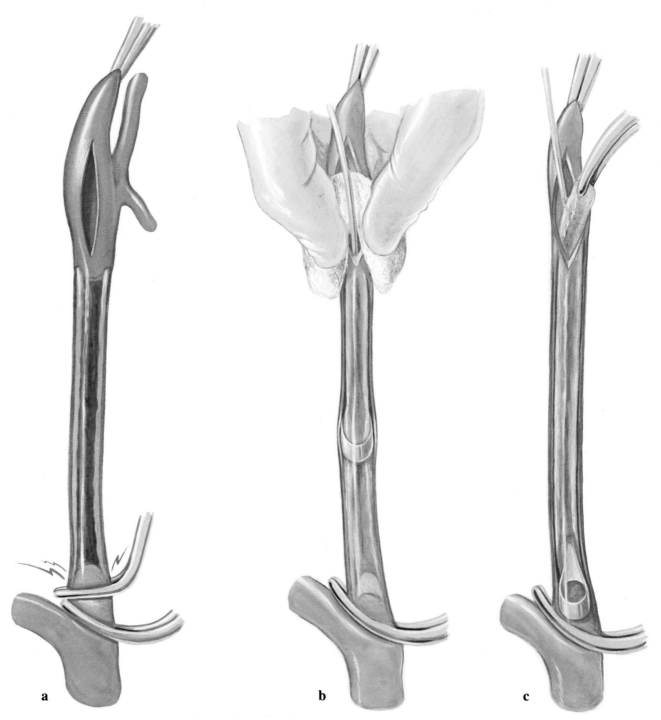

a   b   c

Fig. 3.50,a–c. Closed endarterectomy of right common carotid artery. **a** clamp fracture of proximal intima; **b** retrograde passage of arterial stripper; **c** extraction of intimal core with contained thrombus.

An identical procedure is feasible, but probably not advisable, for left common carotid occlusion. One can generally mobilize the artery through a cervical incision to the level of the aorta without difficulty; however, exposure is not adequate to close an arteriotomy or to repair an inadvertent arterial tear near the common carotid origin. For this reason the endarterectomy is extended to a point just caudal to the clavicle, and the artery is transected at this level. The proximal stump is oversewn, and after re-

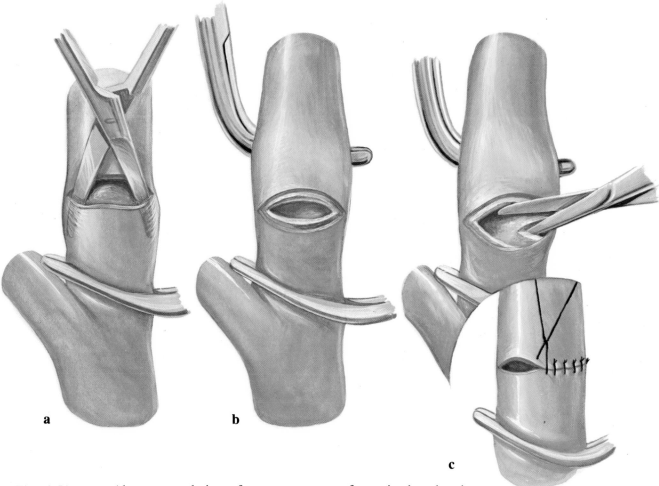

Fig. 3.51,a–c. Alternate technique for management of proximal end point. **a** mobilization of intimal core through a transverse arteriotomy to external surface of the core (stripper has already been passed); **b** incision of core; **c** transection of core and closure of arteriotomy.

moval of the endarterectomy core the distal common carotid artery is transposed laterally and anastomosed end-to-side to the subclavian artery beyond the thyrocervical trunk. The carotid artery should be cut to a length longer than necessary to reach the subclavian artery. Leaving a slightly redundant carotid artery segment allows blood to enter the carotid artery at a 90° angle from its flow direction in the subclavian artery. The artery then assumes a gentle curve behind the sternocleido-mastoid muscle as it returns to its normal position **(Fig. 3.52)**. A shorter carotid segment creates the less favorable acute reversal of flow direction **(Fig. 3.53)**.

This operation is not applicable for patients with associated lesions in the proximal left subclavian artery. Other autogenous tissue reconstructive techniques are available. These include performing a complete carotid endarterectomy to the level of the aorta utilizing a sternotomy approach for control at the proximal end or, as an alternative procedure, through the same incision, transferring the carotid artery to the side of the innominate artery. If there is strong indication for removing the subclavian lesion as well, the entire operation can be performed through a lateral thoractomy approach. After endarterectomy of the subclavian artery the divided left common carotid artery is anastomosed to its side in the mediastinum.

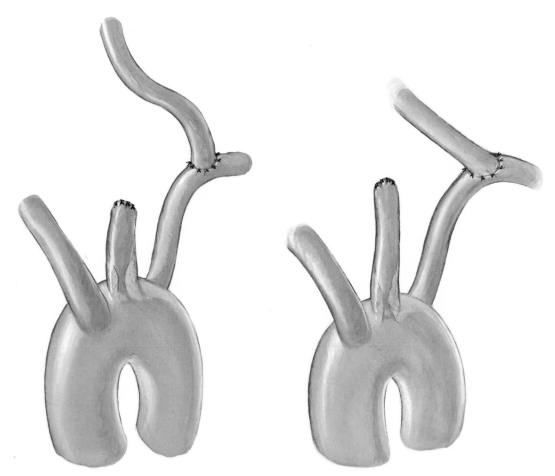

Fig. 3.52. Transfer of left common carotid to left subclavian artery with intentional redundancy of carotid segment.

Fig. 3.53. Undesirable reversal of flow direction with short common carotid segment.

When the internal carotid artery is occluded and the objective of operation is to open the common carotid artery to provide forward flow into the endarterectomized external carotid artery orifice, opening the external carotid artery through a longitudinal arteriotomy to the end of the atherosclerotic lesion is usually necessary to establish an adequate end point. This arteriotomy is closed with a supplementary vein patch.

Atherosclerosis of the Proximal Cervical Arteries

4

Atherosclerosis of the aortic arch branches is usually a multifocal disease with lesions of some degree at the origins of all three branches and in the wall of superior aspect of the aortic arch as well (**Fig. 4.1**). Three general observations are pertinent in defining surgical indications and in the selection of the appropriate operative approach: (1) the extent of individual artery involvement is rarely uniform; (2) except for embolization from the rare ulcerating lesions or progression to occlusion in the case of the left common carotid artery, most of the atherosclerotic lesions at this level do not produce stroke; (3) the collateral channels across the thorax, neck, and face are so voluminous that the net result of single or multiple lesions is often one of symptoms from reduction of total cerebral perfusion rather than of symptoms confined to one area of the brain.

Innominate Lesions

Atherosclerotic lesions in the innominate artery characteristically are most prominent in the proximal one-third of the vessel. The intimal surface may be smooth or grossly ulcerated. When ulceration predominates, its usual location is on the right lateral wall from which it may produce symptoms of distal embolization (usually into the right eye or cerebral hemisphere). As in **Figs. 4.2 and 4.3,** the obstructive lesions usually involve the full circumference at the innominate origin. Stenosis sufficient to impair blood flow will be revealed by a decreased blood pressure in the right arm. Symptoms, if present, are related to decreased cerebral perfusion. Distally, the lesion tends to taper into a posterior plaque that may extend into the posterior wall of the subclavian artery, sparing the common carotid artery. Proximally there is a variable degree of atherosclerotic thickening of the adjacent aortic intima. Rarely the aortic portion of the plaque may extend proximally to within a few centimeters of the pericardial reflection or distally to surround the orifice of the left common carotid artery. A rare variation of this lesion is the accumulation of mural thrombus that may project into the aortic lumen and become the nidus for embolization into the distal branches of the aorta.

The indications for operation are embolization or disabling symptoms secondary to reduced cerebral perfusion. Except for embolizing lesions, atherosclerosis localized to the innominate artery usually does not produce cerebral infarction even when the vessel is occluded.

85

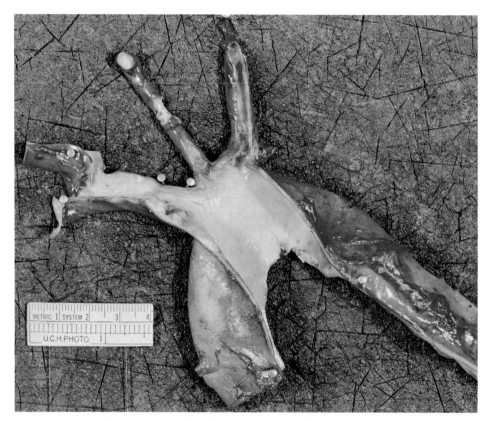

Fig. 4.1. Postmortem specimen of the aortic arch with atherosclerotic lesions at the orifices of the brachiocephalic branches. Lesions occupy the dome of the aortic arch and extend into the proximal 1–2 cm of the three major branches. A discontinuous lesion appears in the left subclavian artery adjacent to the vertebral artery orifice and in the right subclavian artery where the vertebral orifice is only a small fraction of its normal size.

The remaining intimal surface which, at first glance, appears uninvolved has a peculiar succulent consistency. It is thicker than normal and is easily separable by endarterectomy. This pattern of pathologic change is particularly common with atherosclerosis in these arterial segments.

Innominate Endarterectomy

In our own experience the simplest and most satisfactory operation is innominate endarterectomy, a technique that has proved to be durable for maintaining arterial patency and is associated with low morbidity. In-line fabric graft replacement or bypass operations from the ascending aorta are equally durable but introduce the potential complication of perigraft sepsis. Subclavian-to-subclavian crossover grafts create the additional potential of graft thrombosis from turbulence due to the reversal of flow direction at each anastomosis and also the subcutaneous position of the graft. Axillary-to-axillary grafts create an additional problem relative to limitation of shoulder mobility. In 6 out of 34 patients undergoing innominate endarterectomy, the innominate lesion had been the cause of retinal or cerebral emboli. Bypass operations that do not exclude the innominate artery will fail to prevent further embolization.

The low morbidity of a median sternotomy approach has been well established by the thousands of aortocoronary bypass operations using this

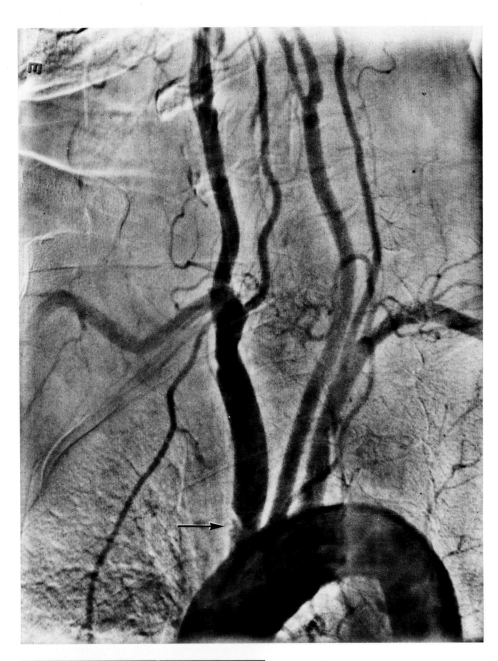

Fig. 4.2. Arch aortogram in a patient with recurrent embolic TEAs to the right hemisphere. Note the ragged ulcerating atherosclerotic lesion at the innominate orifice. Cerebral symptoms ceased following an uncomplicated innominate endarterectomy.

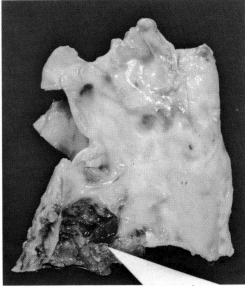

Fig. 4.3. Innominate endarterectomy specimen showing a deep ulcer with contained thrombus at the aortic end.

87

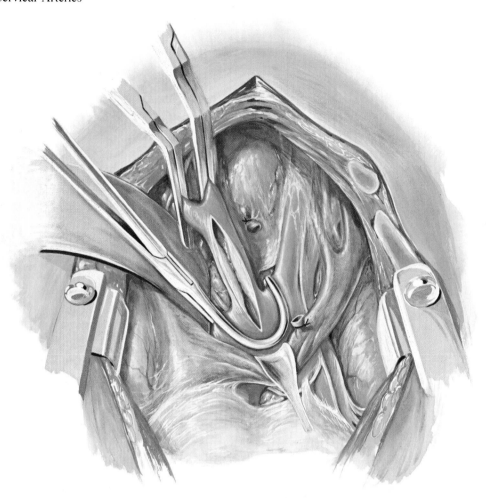

Fig. 4.4. Innominate arteriotomy showing atherosclerotic stenosis of its proximal two-thirds.

approach and has been confirmed by our own experience in innominate reconstruction. **Fig. 4.4** shows the exposure that is developed by this approach. The full length of the sternum has been split. The sternoclavicular attachments have not been disturbed. A specially designed J clamp partially occludes the aorta at the innominate orifice. This must be placed with care to avoid obstruction of the left common carotid artery. Palpation of the aorta before this clamp is applied will reveal the edges of the aortic portion of the atheroma, which usually can be encompassed within the jaws of the clamp. (After application of the proximal clamp it is helpful to measure the pressure in the left common carotid artery to make certain that the clamp has not restricted its orifice to the extent of impairing blood flow to the left hemisphere.) In order to provide ample exposure to deal with the distal end point and to avoid disruption of the mural thrombus which occasionally is attached to the wall of the innominate artery beyond a proximal stenosis, it is desirable to clamp the right common carotid and subclavian arteries individually rather than clamping the distal innominate artery. Before the common carotid artery is clamped for the definitive portion of the operation, its stump pressure is determined. Stump pressures less than the desired 50 mm Hg are rare. Stump pressures substantially less than 50 mm Hg require technique modifications that will be described later (see p. 93).

The longitudinal arteriotomy in the innominate artery is extended into the portion of the aorta within the jaws of the clamp. **Fig. 4.5a** shows the first step in the development of the endarterectomy cleavage plane. The same plane is continued into the wall of the aorta by means of a right-angle clamp, which separates the intima of the aorta to the confines of the J

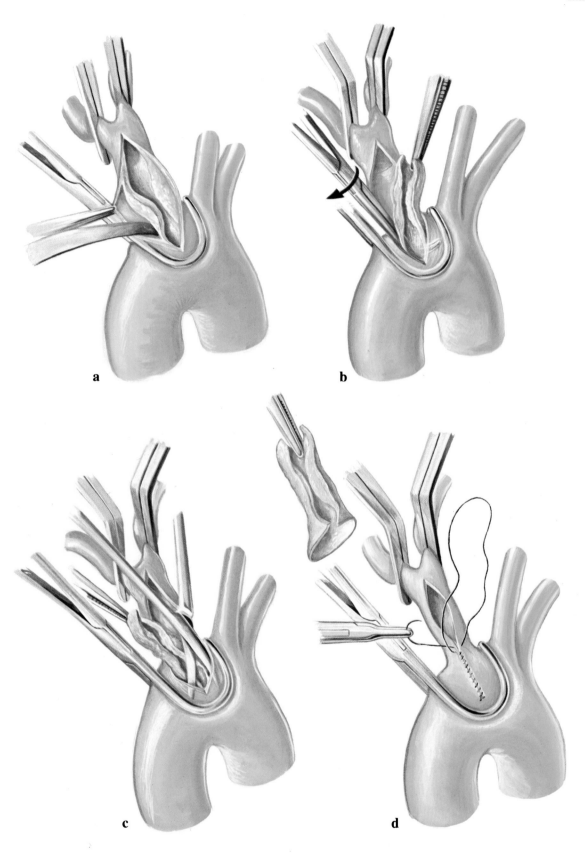

Fig. 4.5,a–d. Steps in innominate endarterectomy. **a** beginning of the dissection plane; **b** development of aortic portion of dissection plane; **c** transection of the aortic intima; **d** closure of the arteriotomy.

clamp (**Fig. 4.5b**). The proximal intimal transection may occasionally be accomplished with scissors inserted beneath the overhanging edges of the aortic media (**Fig. 4.5c**). More often it becomes necessary to extract the partially calcified occluding bolus and residual aortic intimal fragments piecemeal with a curved hemostat. After the usual maneuvers of forward and backward flushing, the arteriotomy is closed with a continuous 4–0 suture (**Fig. 4.5d**). The subclavian and innominate clamps are released first, followed by release of the common carotid clamp. The total time of arterial crossclamping rarely exceeds 15 min. A series of sequential operative photographs of an innominate endarterectomy is shown in **Fig. 4.6a–g.**

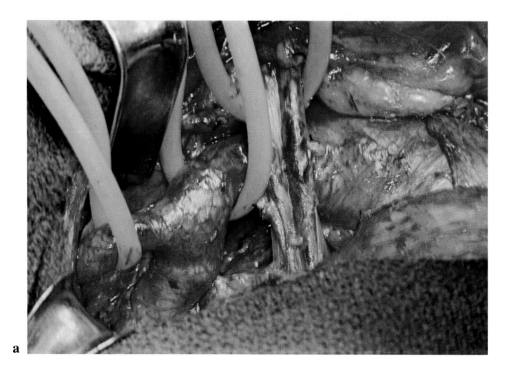

a

Fig. 4.6,a–g. Serial photographs of an innominate endarterectomy in a patient with symptomatic atherosclerotic stenosis at the innominate orifice and palpable extension of disease into the subclavian artery. By palpation the plaque was found to extend into the wall of the aorta adjacent to the innominate origin. **a** The innominate artery, its terminal branches, and the arch of the aorta have been exposed through a sternum-splitting approach. The tubing to the left surrounds the right common carotid artery; the one in the center, the innominate artery; and the one to the right, the innominate vein. The right vagus and recurrent laryngeal nerves are out of view in the lower left. **b** A J clamp partially occludes the aorta and has been placed in a position to surround the aortic portion of the atheroma. Note the yellow color of the aorta in the concavity of the clamp. **c** An arteriotomy has been made from the distal level of palpable disease in the subclavian artery through the full length of the innominate artery and onto the surface of the aorta. The common carotid artery is visible to the left of the upper metal probe. **d** The endarterectomy is started in the midportion of the innominate artery. **e** The mass of atherosclerotic debris in the proximal innominate artery and the adjacent aorta is extracted piecemeal with a hemostat. **f** Except for a few residual tags of tissue that must be removed, the endarterectomy has been completed. **g** After closure of the arteriotomy, circulation is restored first to subclavian artery and finally to the carotid.

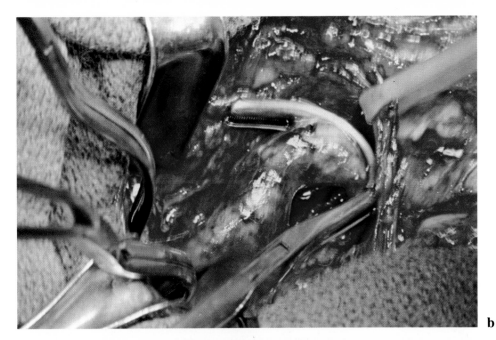

b

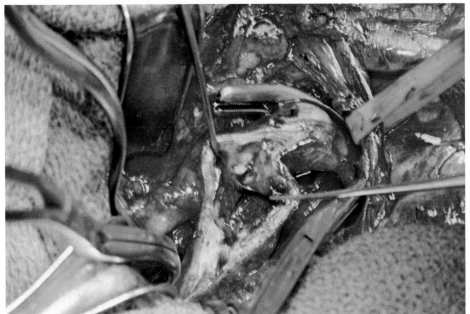

c

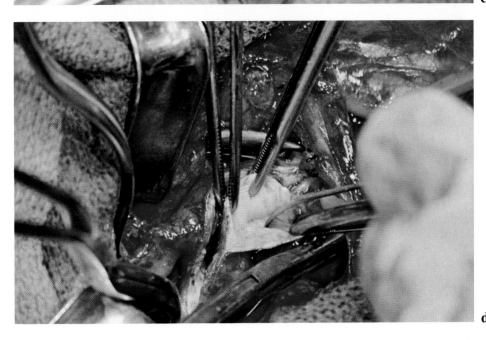

d   **Fig. 4.6** (cont.)

91

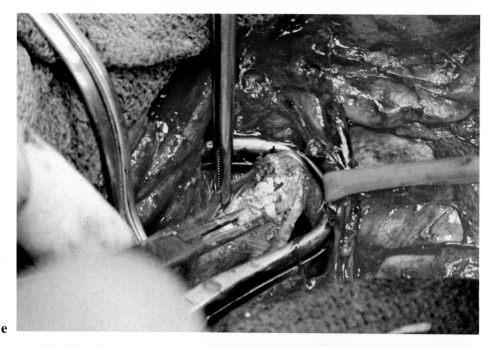

e

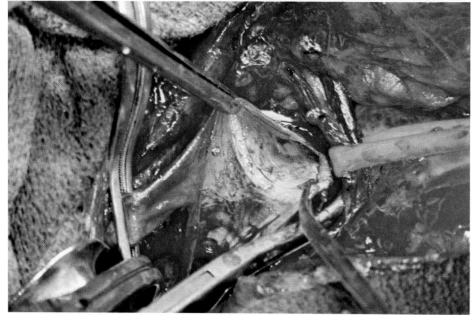

f

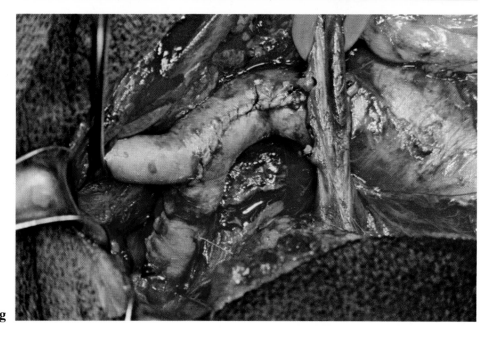

Fig. 4.6 (cont.)

g

92

Bypass Grafts

Bypass grafts are used in the situation where dense atheroma involves the aortic circumference adjacent to the innominate orifice. In this situation, the J clamp is difficult to apply safely and may be inadequate for proximal control. The aortic intima adjacent to the pericardial reflection is usually not involved with atherosclerosis. A partially occluding clamp is applied on the right side of the ascending aorta to provide space for the proximal anastomosis (**Fig. 4.7a**). A knitted, tubular Dacron graft is then placed end-to-side on the aorta and end-to-end to the distal innominate artery (**Fig. 4.7b**).

Maintenance of Cerebral Blood Flow

Fig. 4.8a and b illustrates one technique that may be employed in a patient with an innominate lesion in whom a low carotid stump pressure suggests that common carotid occlusion may not be tolerated without risk of cerebral infarction. A bifurcation graft is anastomosed to the ascending aorta. One limb of this graft is then anastomosed to the subclavian or axillary artery to provide flow into the common carotid artery during the period of distal innominate occlusion. When the other limb has been attached to the innominate artery, the first limb is resected and the stumps oversewn (**Fig. 4.8b**).

Another method for maintaining carotid flow is the use of a temporary T tube internal shunt from the left carotid artery. This is particularly useful in innominate operations where there is a low carotid stump pressure and

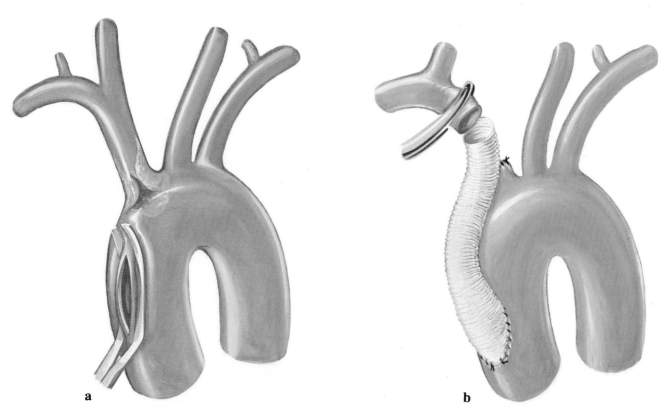

a   b

Fig. 4.7,a, b. Graft replacement of innominate artery. **a** application of partially occluding clamp to side of ascending aorta; **b** preparation for distal anastomosis. The innominate clamp is not applied until the lumen has been inspected and mural thrombus, if present, has been removed.

93

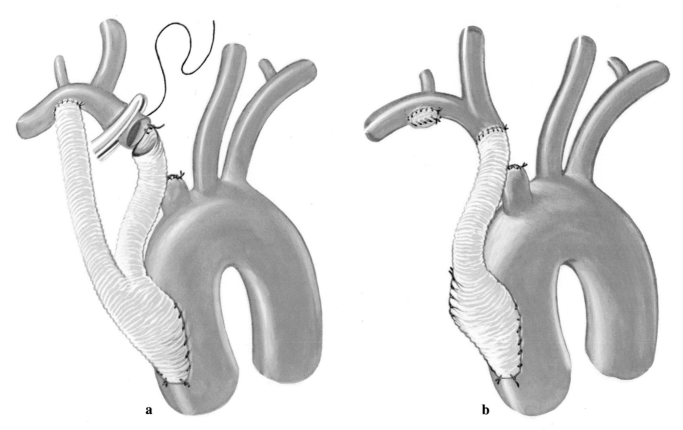

Fig. 4.8,a, b. Grafting technique for preservation of right carotid blood flow. **a** bifurcation graft with temporary limb to subclavian artery; **b** removal of bypass limb after completion of direct anastomosis.

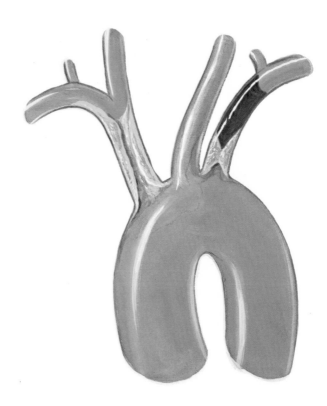

Fig. 4.9. Pathologic situation resulting in inadequate right carotid stump pressure that requires crossover carotid shunt.

the distal extent of the innominate lesion requires clamping of the proximal ipsilateral common carotid artery. This shunting technique is also applicable in another operation when transfer of the left common carotid artery to the left subclavian artery is necessary to bypass a lesion at the left common carotid orifice when collateral blood flow to the left cerebral hemisphere is inadequate to permit temporary clamp occlusion of the carotid artery without a shunt.

A situation in which such a shunt might become necessary is illustrated in **Fig. 4.9.** The distal extension of the innominate lesion makes it necessary to extend the arteriotomy into the subclavian artery, thereby requiring crossclamping of the distal subclavian and the proximal right common carotid arteries. The left subclavian artery is thrombosed, and the only source of cerebral blood supply becomes the left common carotid artery.

In the event that a low right common carotid stump pressure is demonstrated, it becomes necessary to create a temporary shunt from the left common carotid artery that can be inserted rapidly with only momentary interruption of blood flow in the left carotid artery. A T shunt designed for this purpose has been constructed with one arm of the T shorter than the other. A left carotid arteriotomy is made to equal the length of the short arm of the T plus the diameter of the tubing (**Fig. 4.10a**). The long end of the T is inserted first, allowing the short end to fall into the arterial lumen (**Fig. 4.10b**). The shunt is then advanced until the side arm engages the end of the arteriotomy (**Fig. 4.10c**). This provides ample space between the bulbs on the shunt at each end of the arteriotomy for placement of Javid clamps and rapid restoration of blood flow. The shunt now provides blood flow to both hemispheres, allowing time for careful completion of the innominate–subclavian endarterectomy (**Fig. 4.10d**).

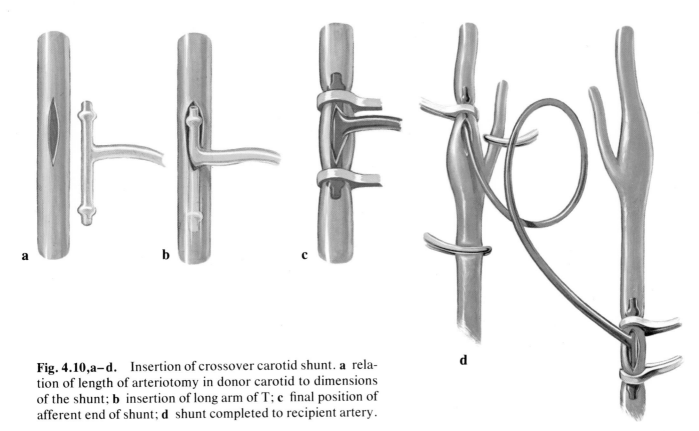

a   b   c

d

Fig. 4.10, a–d. Insertion of crossover carotid shunt. **a** relation of length of arteriotomy in donor carotid to dimensions of the shunt; **b** insertion of long arm of T; **c** final position of afferent end of shunt; **d** shunt completed to recipient artery.

When the shunt is removed, the carotid arteriotomies are closed within the jaws of partially occluding arterial clamps. The only artery in which forward flow has been jeopardized is the right vertebral artery, but we have never encountered a situation in which backbleeding from the vertebral artery has not been vigorous when carotid flow is unimpaired.

Multiple Arch Lesions

Multiple arch lesions require special consideration if revascularization is indicated. Access to all three arteries has generally been considered difficult to obtain safely through either the anterior or left lateral thoracic approaches alone. Revascularization of the left common carotid artery has the greatest priority because of the potential for stroke should it become totally occluded. Transfer of this artery to the left subclavian artery through a cervical approach accomplishes no useful purpose because of the proximal subclavian lesion. Orifice endarterectomy of the left common carotid artery cannot safely be performed through either thoracic route.

If one assumes that dealing simultaneously with the innominate and left common carotid artery accomplishes most of the surgical objectives and that the left subclavian lesion is a benign one if it is the only one remaining, there are two possible techniques that would be applicable in a single operation approached through a median sternotomy. One would be the placement of a bifurcation graft from the side of the ascending aorta with branches to the common carotid artery on the left and on the right to the distal innominate or the proximal right subclavian or common carotid arteries, whichever is most suitable. The other method would be to open the innominate artery by endarterectomy and to extend a small tubular graft from either the side of the aorta or the side of the innominate artery to the left common carotid artery.

The latter technique has several advantages over the former. It is generally simpler to find a suitable donor area and to create an anastomosis to the side of the aorta for a small 6-mm graft than the larger aortic end of a bifurcation graft. A single small tubular graft lessens the sheer bulk of fabric material in the superior mediastinum and thereby reduces the risk of infection. Finally, extension of the innominate endarterectomy incision allows one to deal directly with the frequently contiguous lesions in the right subclavian and right vertebral arteries.

Fig. 4.11a and b shows the pre- and postoperative aortograms of a combined endarterectomy and grafting operation. **Fig. 4.12a–c** shows the preoperative aortogram and an operative photograph of another patient with the same operation.

Recent experiences have shown that safe access to the proximal left subclavian artery is technically feasible through the anterior sternotomy approach in many patients. Although not applicable for endarterectomy, this approach enables one to bring a graft from the ascending aorta for an end-to-end anastomosis to the left subclavian artery distal to an orifice lesion within it. When multiple arch branch lesions are present and collateral flow is scanty, the use of this graft as the first reconstructive step provides forward flow into the left vertebral artery. In our experience this maneuver alone may double the stump pressures in the other arch branches and remove the necessity for temporary shunting procedures.

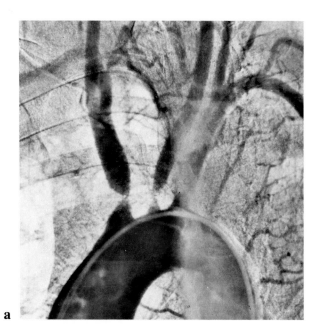
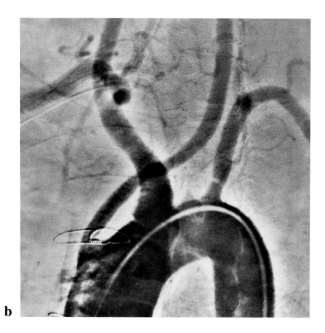

a

b

Fig. 4.11,a, b. Preoperative (**a**) and postoperative (**b**) arch aortograms of a 45-year-old male with severe stenosis at the orifices of the innominate and left common carotid arteries and a lesser lesion in the left subclavian artery. At operation the individual stump pressures in the innominate and the left common carotid arteries exceeded 50 mm Hg but when measured while the other artery was occluded dropped to less than 30 mm Hg.

The lesion in the innominate artery was removed by endarterectomy. A 6-mm flanged Dacron graft (cut from a 12 × 6 bifurcation graft) was anastomosed proximally to the side of the ascending aorta and distally end-to-end to the transected left common carotid artery. Access to the left subclavian artery is also possible through this exposure, but in this case revascularization of the left subclavian artery was considered to be unnecessary. In the unlikely event that the residual left subclavian lesion ever becomes symptomatic, this will be dealt with by either a left transthoracic endarterectomy or a carotid–subclavian graft or transposition operation in the neck.

Vertebrosubclavian Atherosclerosis

The primary objective of operations for atherosclerosis in the subclavian or vertebral arteries is the relief of symptoms of vertebrobasilar insufficiency. Obstructing lesions at these sites, in the absence of obstruction in the carotid system, rarely cause infarction in the vertebrobasilar territory. Symptoms of decreased vertebrobasilar perfusion may be sufficiently disabling, however, to require operation for their relief. The most common are episodic visual loss, diplopia, ataxia, or drop attacks. The classical alternating long-tract symptoms of basilar insufficiency are usually the result of primary lesions in the basilar artery or its branches, currently surgically approachable only by extracranial–intracranial bypass operations. The symptom of giddiness, at one time considered diagnostic of vertebrobasilar insufficiency, appears to be nonspecific and often appears with carotid occlusive disease as well.

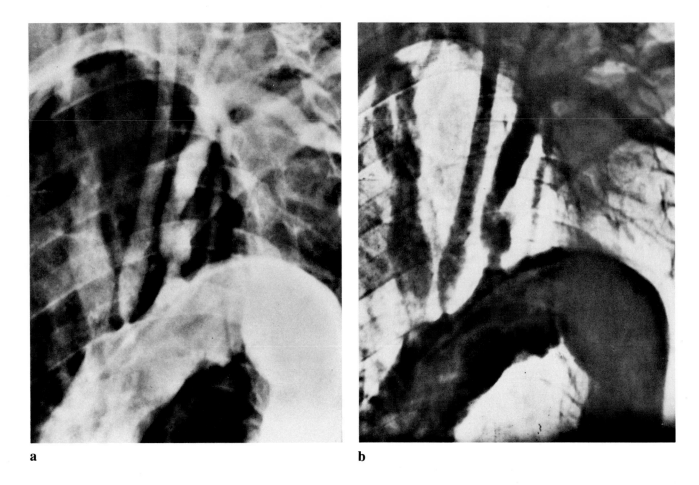

a

b

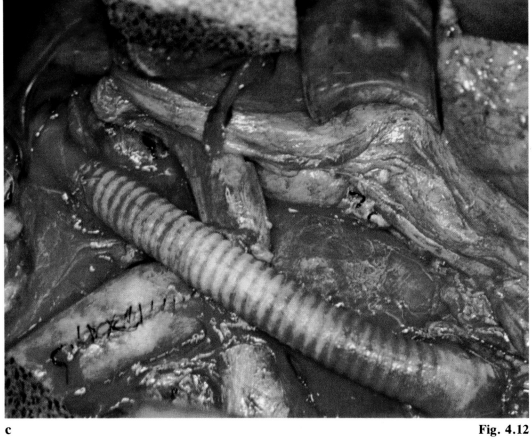

c

Fig. 4.12

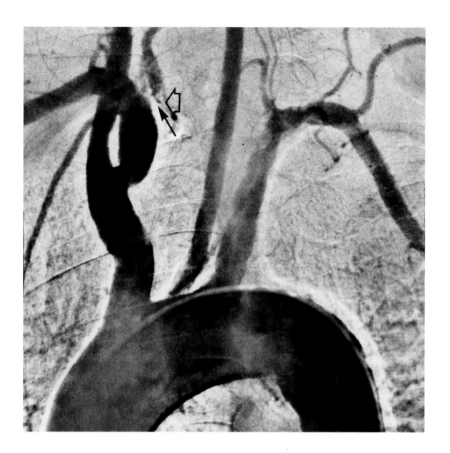

Fig. 4.13. Arch aortogram in a patient with symptoms of vertebrobasilar insufficiency secondary to atherosclerotic stenosis of the right vertebral artery and occlusion of the left. The bilateral pattern of disease is a characteristic distribution when symptoms are the result of disease or anomalies in the proximal segments of the vertebrobasilar system.

Two anatomic considerations influence the decision for operation when vertebral or subclavian artery lesions have been demonstrated. First, carotid stenosis, if present, may substantially impair collateral flow to the vertebrobasilar territory. A successful operation on the carotid arteries will often relieve the symptoms of ischemia in the posterior circulation and eliminate the need for vertebral–subclavian reconstruction. Although residual lesions may progress to complete occlusion, cerebral infarction rarely results. Second, symptoms of vertebrobasilar insufficiency, as a result of pure vertebral or subclavian artery disease, develop only when flow in *both* vertebral arteries is impaired (**Fig. 4.13**). Bilateral

---

Fig. 4.12,a–c Arch aortograms (**a and b**) in a patient with atherosclerotic stenosis of the three brachiocephalic branches. Severe stenosis of the innominate orifice was revealed by the lesser density visible only in the subtraction film (**b**).

The flattening of the aortic arch is the result of a lengthy atheroma in the dome of the arch. Revascularization needs are limited to the innominate and the almost-occluded left common carotid artery. The lesion in the left subclavian artery makes this an inadequate afferent artery for a transposition or grafting operation to restore normal forward flow in the left carotid artery.

c At operation, a small area of undiseased aortic wall could be palpated in the ascending aorta adequate in size for the attachment of a 6-mm graft. This graft was anastomosed end-to-end to the left common carotid. The atheroma in the innominate artery and the adjacent aorta was removed by the conventional innominate endarterectomy technique.

At the conclusion of procedures (patient's head is to the left), the proximal graft anastomosis in the right lower corner is to the ascending aorta at the distal level of the locally resected pericardial reflection. The partial compression of the innominate vein was not associated with increase in proximal venous pressure. The innominate artery can be identified as the artery with the suture line in the arteriotomy.

impairment of vertebral flow may occur as a result of any combination of vertebral and proximal subclavian artery disease, or with unilateral vertebral obstruction when the contralateral vertebral artery is hypoplastic. Stenosis of one vertebral or subclavian artery rarely causes vertebrobasilar ischemia if the contralateral subclavian and vertebral arteries are of normal size. The only exception occurs in the congenital variant, where one vertebral artery terminates in the posterior inferior cerebellar artery rather than the basilar artery.

Subclavian stenosis or occlusion only rarely produces symptomatic ischemia of the arm. Collateral circulation to the arm is abundant, and except for patients with occupational requirements for normal blood flow (e.g., carpenters), limb ischemia with exercise is negligible. The once-popular concept that arm exercise in the presence of a proximal subclavian occlusion (with reversal of blood flow in the ipsilateral vertebral artery) results in basilar ischemia has received scant support from clinical observations. The only situations we have encountered in which subclavian lesions result in substantial limb ischemia have been when a previous operation has destroyed the cervical collateral branches or when the ipsilateral vertebral artery is also occluded. Limb ischemia may also occur when the primary lesion is ulcerated and has produced multiple emboli to the arm. This latter event has occurred in our experience only with atherosclerosis at the orifice of the left subclavian artery or when embolization has occurred from a mural thrombus within a poststenotic subclavian aneurysm in a patient with a cervical rib.

The common cause of chronic vertebral stenosis or occlusion is atherosclerosis. Compression from osteophytes in the cervical vertebrae and arteritis are two additional, but rare, causes. Ligamentous bands across the proximal portions of the artery have been reported, but we have never encountered them. Atherosclerotic lesions in the vertebral arteries are confined to the proximal 1–2 cm. They have an abrupt end point beyond which the intima is thin and firmly attached and are associated with variable degrees of atherosclerosis in the subclavian artery adjacent to the vertebral orifice.

The common obstructing lesion of subclavian atherosclerosis commonly presents on the right side as an atheromatous diaphragm adjacent to the innominate artery. Rarely does the subclavian lesion have the abrupt end point seen in carotid lesions, and particular care must be taken to prevent a distal flap during operation. On both sides the atherosclerotic lesion may be confined to the intima surrounding the vertebral orifice or may be associated with extensive subclavian disease proximal and, rarely, distal to it.

The right subclavian artery rises to a higher level in the neck than does the left. Atherosclerotic lesions in the right subclavian and vertebral arteries are effectively removed by endarterectomy. Exposure through a supraclavicular cervical approach is usually adequate. Only rarely is it necessary to use a median sternotomy incision. Either approach is preferable to the cosmetically disfiguring technique of resecting the head of the clavicle.

The cervical incision for approach to the right vertebral and subclavian arteries and the anatomy in the lower cervical triangle is illustrated in **Fig. 4.14a and b.** The origin of the vertebral artery lies behind the jugular vein. Access to the vertebral artery requires division of the clavicular head of the sternocleidomastoid and the scalenus anticus muscles.

The jugular vein is retracted laterally to allow exposure for a longitudinal arteriotomy in the subclavian artery (**Fig. 4.15a and b**). The wall of

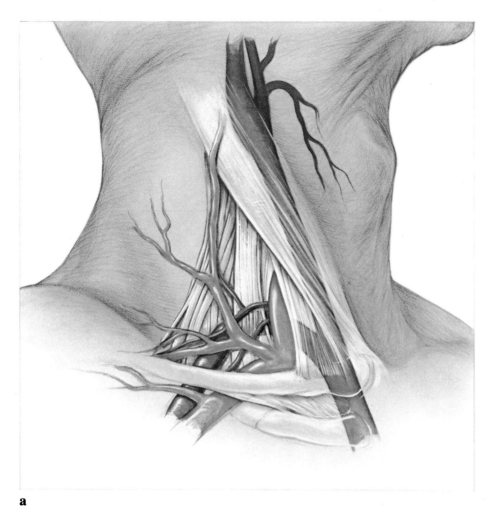

a

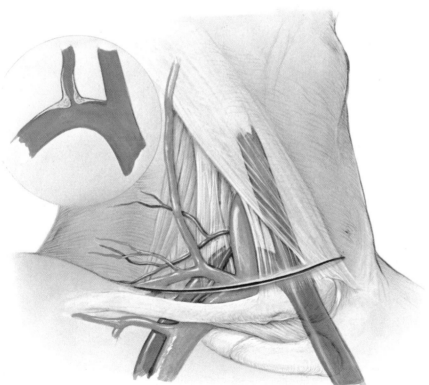

b

Fig. 4.14,a, b. Approach to right subclavian and vertebral arteries. **a** anatomy of posterior triangle of the neck; **b** skin incision and structures adjacent to vertebral orifice with drawing of characteristic pattern of atherosclerotic lesion at the vertebral orifice (**inset**).

101

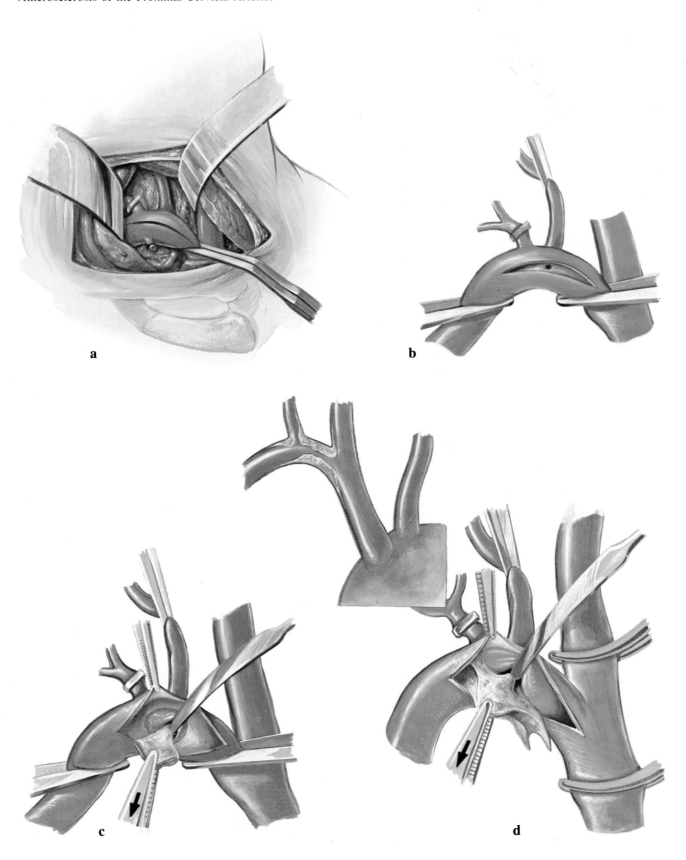

Fig. 4.15,a–d. Transsubclavian technique for vertebral endarterectomy. **a** longitudinal subclavian arteriotomy centered at vertebral artery; **b** stenosed vertebral orifice visible in opposite wall of subclavian artery; **c** removal of vertebral lesion with disc of adjacent subclavian intima; **d** combined subclavian and vertebral endarterectomy.

the subclavian artery is unusually fragile, and particular care must be taken to prevent lateral tears at the end of the arteriotomy. When the vertebral lesion is associated with only minimal involvement of the subclavian artery, a local endarterectomy is adequate. A circumferential incision is made into the subclavian intima surrounding the vertebral orifice. An endarterectomy plane is then developed into the wall of the vertebral artery until the end point is reached (**Fig. 4.15c**). The specimen is easily detached without disturbing the normal distal intima.

 If, as often happens, one encounters substantial disease in the subclavian artery, a sleeve of subclavian intima should be removed to include the orifice lesion in the vertebral artery (**Fig. 4.15d**). A sharply defined end point in the subclavian artery may be difficult to establish, and tack-down sutures may become necessary. With this technique there is no need for a supplemental patch graft angioplasty since after the clamps have been released, the endarterectomized segment of the vertebral artery will distend to a greater than normal diameter. The clip on the thyrocervical trunk in Fig. 4.15 will be removed at completion of the operation. As with any operation on an atherosclerotic subclavian artery as many branches as possible are preserved to be available as collateral to the arm in the rare event of later subclavian occlusion.

 Safe access to the left subclavian artery for vertebral endarterectomy by the same technique can only rarely be accomplished by a cervical approach. A simple and durable cervical operation is to transpose the vertebral artery to the side of the left common carotid artery (**Fig. 4.16**). It is advisable to mobilize the vertebral artery to the point of its entrance into the osseous canal at C_6 level. Transsubclavian endarterectomy is a satisfactory alternate technique, but requires a left thoracotomy and is used only when associated proximal subclavian artery disease requires attention.

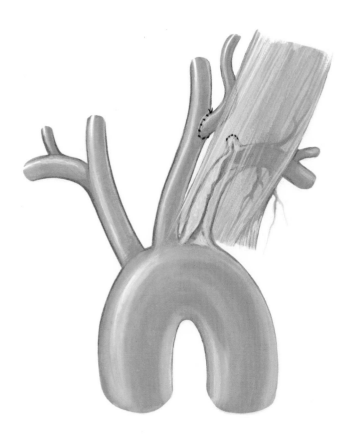

Fig. 4.16. Transposition of left vertebral artery to left common carotid.

103

As with innominate stenosis, the subclavian lesion often extends into the adjacent wall of the aorta. **Figs. 4.17 and 4.18** illustrate one of the first operative techniques used for left subclavian stenosis or occlusion, i.e., transthoracic subclavian endarterectomy. The chest is opened through a 3rd interspace anterolateral thoracotomy (Fig. 4.17). A specially designed J clamp is applied to the aorta to surround the aortic portion of the atheroma. Endarterectomy is performed through a longitudinal arteriotomy (Fig. 4.18). Atherosclerosis in the vertebral orifice, if present, is managed

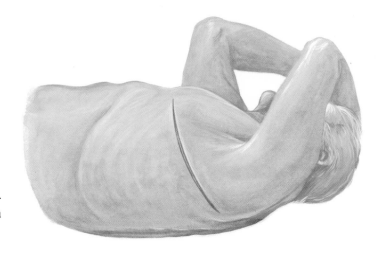

Fig. 4.17. Incision for transthoracic approach to left subclavian and vertebral arteries.

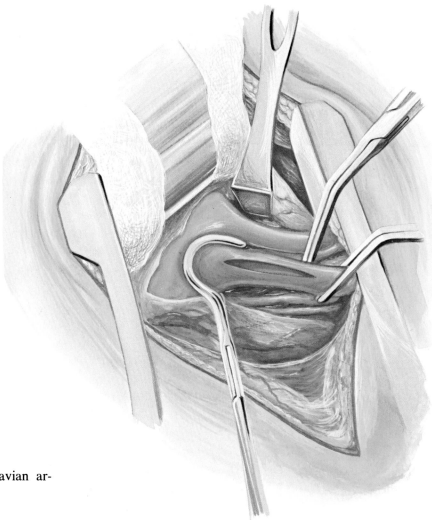

Fig. 4.18. Left subclavian arteriotomy.

by the same technique used for right vertebral stenosis. The only disadvantage of this technique is the potentially greater morbidity caused by the thoracotomy. With the passage of time this operation is proving to be more durable than the cervical bypass techniques, and for this reason has become the preferred technique except for the rare patient for whom thoracotomy introduces a prohibitive risk.

Fig. 4.19 shows the commonly employed bypass graft from the common carotid artery to the distal subclavian artery. In this illustration a saphenous vein segment has been used. (**Fig. 4.20** is an operative photograph of a saphenous vein in place.) The long-term attrition rate of a saphenous

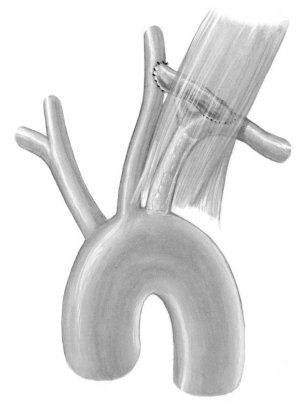

Fig. 4.19. Carotid subclavian bypass graft (using saphenous vein).

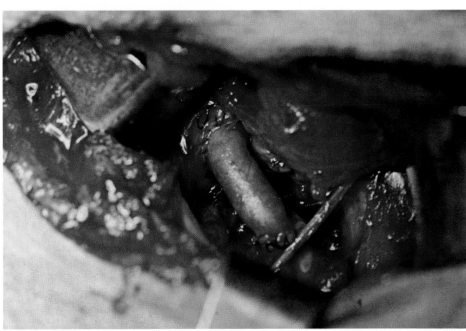

Fig. 4.20. Saphenous vein graft from the side of the left common carotid artery to the left subclavian artery in a patient with symptoms of vertebrobasilar insufficiency secondary to occlusion of the right vertebral and the left subclavian arteries.

105

vein placed in the arterial circuit is now recognized, and one can expect a predictable frequency of late failure. Dacron grafts used in this situation are more durable but introduce new problems should perigraft sepsis develop.

The use of bypass grafts alone is, of course, an unacceptable technique for the management of embolizing lesions in the proximal subclavian artery. When embolization has occurred in a patient whose general condition prohibits transthoracic endarterectomy to remove the lesion, isolation of the lesion can usually be accomplished by transposing the subclavian artery (transected distal to the lesion) to the side of the common carotid artery (**Fig. 4.21**). Although this procedure is more easily accomplished by a thoracic approach, it can also be performed through a cervical incision.

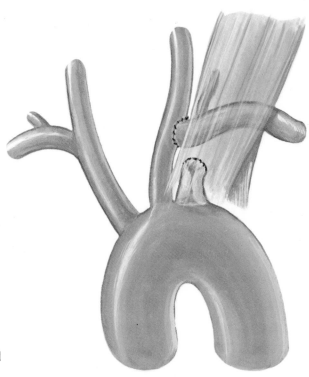

Fig. 4.21. Subclavian–carotid transposition.

Aortoiliac Atherosclerosis

5

Patterns of Atherosclerosis

The natural history of the developing pathology of atherosclerosis in the aorta and iliac arteries is a major factor in the selection of the most appropriate and durable surgical technique when operation becomes indicated.

Abdominal Aorta

Obstructive intimal lesions tend to appear first in the region of the aortic bifurcation and involve one or both of the common iliac arteries and both of the hypogastric arteries. By this time, a lesser degree of intimal disease will be present in the more proximal aorta to at least the level of the renal arteries. Disease in this segment almost inevitably progresses and, in time, becomes genuinely obstructive.

Variations in the pattern of development of occlusive atherosclerosis in the abdominal aorta are occasionally encountered. In one, the entire length of the subdiaphragmatic abdominal aorta becomes involved simultaneously with marked, diffuse intimal thickening. The intimal surface, although irregular, maintains a smooth surface and, when resected, has an almost rubbery consistency. The intimal thickening appears to overflow the orifices of the branching arteries. Although intimal thickening in the more distal portions of the aorta may be more advanced, patients with this form of aortic atherosclerosis frequently are first seen because of renovascular hypertension or chronic visceral ischemia.

In another form of the disease, typical occlusive lesions may be confined to the region of the aortic bifurcation, but the aortic intima in the segment between the superior and inferior mesenteric arteries will have undergone necrotic, amorphous, granular degeneration without substantial narrowing of the aortic lumen. Although often not apparent on the aortogram, this condition creates a genuine hazard when an aortic operation is performed.

Rarely the occlusive lesion may appear first in the aortic segment between the renal and the inferior mesenteric arteries. The aortogram may suggest that the distal aorta and the iliac arteries are free of disease. At operation, however, distal disease to at least the level of the common iliac bifurcations is palpable and must be dealt with in planning a durable operation.

A more common pattern in the development of aortic occlusion to the level of the renal arteries is the result of proximal propagation of thrombus from a totally occluding atherosclerotic lesion in the distal infrarenal segment (see figure below). Continuing proximal propagation of thrombus in time will occlude the renal orifices. The aortographic demonstration of occlusion at the subrenal level thus presents a stronger indication for operation than atherosclerosis at more distal levels.

Iliac Arteries

Distally the disease takes one of two separate forms. The less extensive (and the less common) is one in which atherosclerosis remains confined to the infrarenal aorta, the common iliac, the hypogastric, and the first 1–2 cm of the external iliac arteries. For purposes of later reference, we will label this *type A disease*. Patients with this form of the disease may live for years before they develop disease in the distal external iliac and femoral arteries.

In the other form of the disease, *type B,* spotty or continuous posterior intimal thickening in the full length of the external iliac arteries will be present almost from the onset. These lesions are inevitably progressive and are usually associated with similar lesions in the common and superficial femoral arteries and to a variable degree in the orifices of the profunda femoris arteries. The last artery to become extensively diseased is the profunda femoris artery, and when this occurs, involvement is usually limited to the first 8–10 cm. Regardless of which of the two patterns of distal disease is encountered, the pattern of common or external iliac disease that may at first seem unilateral eventually becomes bilateral.

In most patients with occlusive atherosclerosis, the gross pathologic changes are confined to the intima. The media retains its normal appearance and strength. However, the interlamellar bands of the media in a zone near the media–intima interface become weakened. It is in this zone that a dissection plane can be developed to perform an endarterectomy. In an occasional patient with aortoiliac obstructive lesions, the media will have undergone more extensive destruction with weakening of the entire wall, primarily in the aortic segment (**Fig. 5.1**). At operation, the aorta appears patulous and irregularly and perceptibly widened. An aorta with this type of atherosclerosis eventually culminates in frank aneurysm.

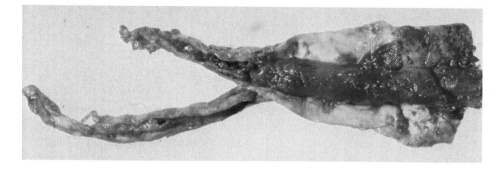

Fig. 5.1. Endarterectomy specimen in a patient with occlusion of the entire infrarenal aorta and the common iliac arteries. The occlusive portion of the atherosclerotic lesion was confined to the common iliac arteries. The aorta has become occluded by proximal progression of thrombosis to the level of the renal arteries. Note the tongue of atheroma that has been removed from the left external iliac artery.

The clinical objective of arterial reconstruction in most patients with aortoiliac atherosclerosis is the relief of claudication. In patients with type A disease, walking tolerances may vary from 200 to 1000 m (usually expressed by the patient in terms of city blocks). Many of these patients are relatively young (age range: 35–55 years), and their fairly mild degree of claudication may be a genuinely functional impairment. The lesions are not limb threatening, however, and the indication for operation is based solely on the degree of functional incapacity. The only exception to this statement occurs in the patients whose aortic occlusion has ascended to the infrarenal level and who are vulnerable to renal arterial blood flow impairment from proximal propagation of thrombus.

In the patients with type B disease, extensive involvement of the external iliac and/or common femoral arteries causes a much greater and often intolerable restriction in walking tolerance. If the profunda and superficial femoral arteries have retained their patency, the more severe forms of ischemia, i.e., rest pain and tissue necrosis, are uncommon.

Patients with type B disease are more vulnerable, however, to future limb-threatening complications than are those with type A disease. Some degree of atherosclerosis in the superficial femoral arteries is usually present and, in time, progresses to total occlusion. Collateral flow in the profunda femoris artery has already been reduced by the proximal obstructive lesions. Operation for limb salvage then often becomes necessary. Restoration of normal flow into the profunda circuit, unless there are advanced lesions at the popliteal trifurcation, will usually return the patient to the state of mild claudication that can be anticipated from the residual superficial femoral artery occlusion. This degree of claudication is usually well tolerated. There is, of course, a potential for future recurrence of severe ischemia if a residual stenosing lesion is allowed to remain in the proximal profunda artery. Later closure of this artery nullifies the gain obtained from the aortofemoral reconstructive operation.

Principles in Selection of Operation

From the foregoing, certain principles in the selection of the most appropriate operation for either type A or B aortoiliac disease and precautions in their performance can be listed:

1. The proximal end of a revascularization operation, whether it be bypass or endarterectomy, should be in the portion of the aorta as close as possible to the renal arteries. To begin the reconstruction at a more distal level invites recurrence of symptoms as disease progresses in the proximal unoperated segment.
2. The primary operation, except under unusual circumstances, should be bilateral. A unilateral operation for apparent unilateral iliac disease will be followed, in time, by symptoms on the other side as the bilateral pattern of disease becomes established.
3. When any degree of external iliac disease is palpable beyond the first 1–2 cm, the operation should be extended to the groins.
4. In the type B pattern of disease, the ultimate objective is the development of normal blood flow into the profunda femoris arteries and their distal branches. Since these generally are the last portions of the major arterial segments beyond the groins to become atherosclerotic, they ultimately become the outflow vessels of a proximal reconstructed segment and the collateral supply to the lower legs in the event of present

109

or subsequent occlusion of the superficial femoral arteries. Thus, if proximal profunda lesions are encountered, profundaplasty should be included as a part of the operation.

5. Extreme care should be utilized in mobilizing the aorta for either bypass or endarterectomy. Excessive manipulation of the aorta may cause distal embolic occlusions.

6. The release of aortic clamps after completion of the aortic anastomosis in a bypass operation should be done while the external iliac arteries are temporarily occluded to flush loose aortic intimal fragments into the pelvis via the hypogastric vessels.

7. A patulous aorta in a patient with occlusive symptoms should be resected in the same manner as for an aortic aneurysm.

Endarterectomy

Advantages

Endarterectomy was the first technique introduced for the treatment of aortoiliac atherosclerosis. This method has two major advantages over bypass techniques. One, it is an autogenous tissue technique and is, therefore, less vulnerable to infection. We have never encountered a situation where sepsis after aortoiliac endarterectomy failed to resolve or caused arterial disruption. Second, when sexual impotence has occurred because of disease proximal to or within the hypogastric arteries, endarterectomy has the potential for restoring potency (30% in our own experience). It is important to note, however, that although normal penile erection and orgasm may be restored, forward ejaculation will often be lost. Restoration of potency should not be the sole indication for revascularization operation on the abdominal aorta.

Disadvantages

There are two disadvantages of endarterectomy when compared to bypass operations. One is the vulnerability of an endarterectomized artery to recurrent atherosclerosis. Although the frequency of this as a clinical problem is low (less than 1.5% per year beginning after the third year in the follow-up period), it is important to recognize that a fabric graft is essentially immune to this complication. Although evaluation of this disadvantage in the perspective of published data suggests that late failure of bypass grafts is no less frequent, the causes of late graft occlusion are likely to be more iatrogenic than biologic.

The second disadvantage of endarterectomy is the greater skill and experience that is required for mastery of the technique. At the time of this writing, the number of patients in whom aortoiliac endarterectomy is feasible exceeds by far the number of surgeons who have had the opportunity to become familiar with this technique. Aortoiliac endarterectomy in the hands of an inexperienced surgeon is more prone to immediate failure than is a bypass procedure performed by the same surgeon.

Some surgeons have cited two further contraindications to endarterectomy that have not been supported by our own experience. One is that it is a technique suitable only for short lesions and is apt to fail when more lengthy lesions are encountered. For reasons cited previously, endarterectomy in our hands always includes at least the full length of the infrarenal aorta and both common iliac arteries. These operations, and even longer ones, extended throughout the full length of both external iliac and common femoral arteries function as well as if a prosthetic graft had been used.

The other frequently cited contraindication is mural calcification. Although occasionally calcification in the aorta may create circumferential rigidity comparable to that of a metal pipe, calcification occurs only in the layer that is normally removed by operation. The uninvolved media retains its normal strength. In many situations, however, calcification may make inserting the sutures for a bypass operation impossible, and endarterectomy becomes the only technically feasible procedure. In the situation where circumferential calcification extends to the level of the renal arteries, it may become necessary to temporarily crossclamp the aorta cephalad to the renal arteries (a zone usually free of calcification) while the proximal portion of the endarterectomy is being performed. The customary endarterectomy plane may often be developed without attempting to enter the aortic lumen. When calcification is circumferential, the endarterectomy specimen at the proximal end may often require a bone rongeur for its removal.

Contraindications

The one pathologic situation that does constitute a contraindication to endarterectomy is the presence of preaneurysmal degeneration of the aortic wall, which can readily be recognized by irregular zones of aortic dilatation. Medial degeneration extends more deeply into the aortic wall. The customary dissection plane may be developed without difficulty but the strength of the remaining medial layer is inadequate to resist permanently the intraluminal pressure and the late (5–10 years) appearance of a frank aneurysm can be anticipated.

Operative Technique

Figures 5.2–5.12 show the steps in the performance of aortailiac endarterectomy in a patient with *type A distribution of atherosclerosis*. The desirability of extending the aortic portion of the endarterectomy to the level of the renal arteries and the demands for unimpeded exposure of the common iliac bifurcations, the hypogastric arteries, and the proximal portions of the external iliac arteries make it necessary to use a full-length longitudinal incision in the abdominal wall. Although the preoperative aortograms may have suggested that the external iliac arteries are free of atherosclerosis, the final determination requires careful palpation to the level of the inguinal ligaments. Scattered or lengthy lesions, usually situated in the posterior wall of the external iliac arteries, can often be detected by palpation in the iliac fossae through the intact peritoneum. If lesions are present in any degree, the reconstructive operation must be extended to the groins. If, in this case, the alternative operation of aortofemoral bypass is selected, the extensive retroperitoneal exposure described below is unnecessary.

The retroperitoneal incision on the surface of the aorta is placed slightly to the right of the midline and is extended onto the anterior surface of the right common iliac artery in order to avoid the inferior mesenteric artery and its sigmoidal branches **(Fig. 5.2)**. The incision should be deepened immediately to the aortic adventitia to permit skeletonization of the aorta in this plane without interrupting the preaortic sympathetic fibers. Particular attention is paid to preserving the bundle of nerve fibers crossing the proximal left common iliac artery as they descend into the pelvis. Transection of these fibers is believed to be one cause of postoperative sexual

111

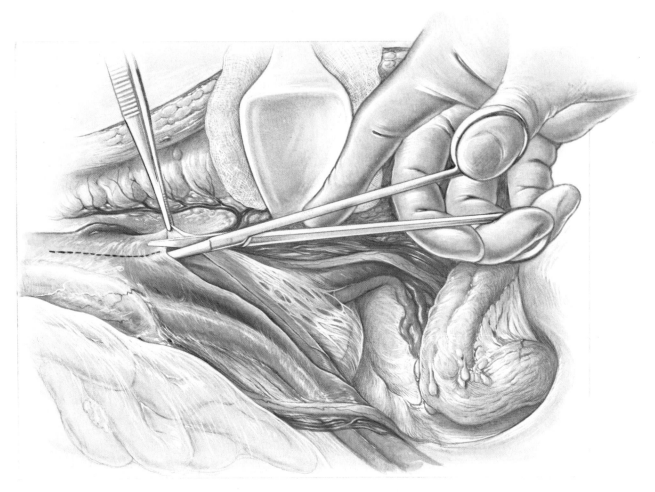

Fig. 5.2. Posterior peritoneal incision.

impotence. For clarity of exposition these fibers are not shown in the subsequent drawings.

Complete but atraumatic mobilization of the aorta is a critical phase of the operation. The degree of friable intimal degeneration usually greatly exceeds that which one might anticipate from the aortographic picture, and distal embolization is a constant threat. **Fig. 5.3a and b** shows the precautions being used to avoid disturbing the aorta. Tunnels are developed between successive pairs of lumbar arteries with the finger pressed firmly against the vertebrae (**Fig. 5.3c**).

Lumbar sympathectomy has become a routine in all of our intra-abdominal operations for arterial occlusive disease. This is limited to a single ganglionectomy on each side, usually at the L-3 level (**Fig. 5.4**). A more extensive sympathectomy is unnecessary and increases the frequency of postsympathectomy neuralgia.

The proper extent of endarterectomy for type A disease, regardless of the extent of gross disease, is from the aorta at the level of the renal arteries through the full length of both common iliac arteries. The endarterectomy includes the usually present tongue of thickened intima in the first 1–2 cm of the external iliac arteries and is extended, if possible, to the end of the hypogastric artery lesions.

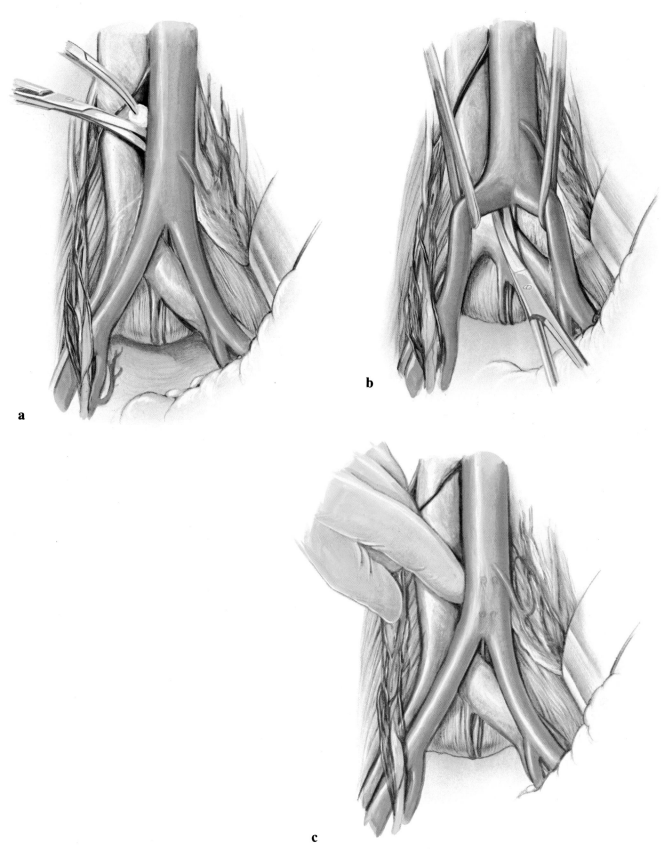

Fig. 5.3,a–c. Skeletonization of aorta and iliac arteries. **a** dissection without aortic retraction (preserved preiliac nerve plexus not shown); **b** posterior dissection of aortic bifurcation; **c** creation of tunnels between successive pairs of lumbar arteries with finger or instrumental probing.

113

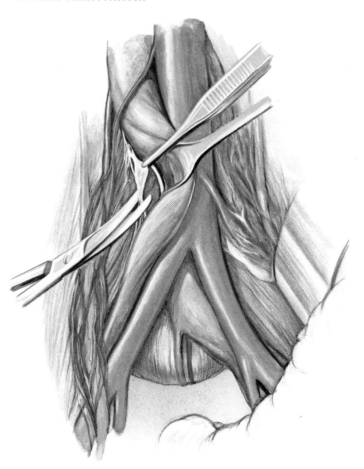

Fig. 5.4. Resection of L-3 sympathetic ganglion.

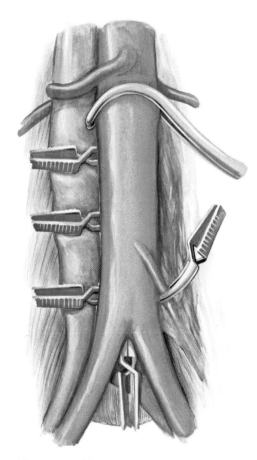

Fig. 5.5. Clamps in place.

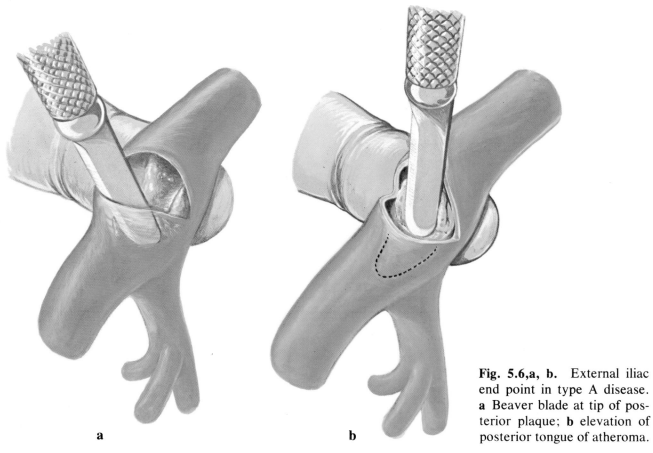

a

b

Fig. 5.6,a, b. External iliac end point in type A disease. **a** Beaver blade at tip of posterior plaque; **b** elevation of posterior tongue of atheroma.

114

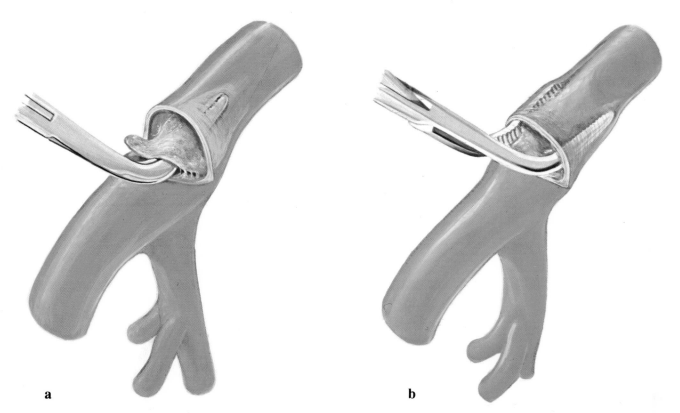

a   b

Fig. 5.7,a, b. Development of atheromatous core in common iliac artery.
a proximal insertion of angled clamp; **b** clamp jaws spread.

Fig. 5.5 shows the aortic clamp in place with bulldog clamps on the lumbar and inferior mesenteric arteries. Clamps have also been placed on the external iliac arteries distal to palpable disease and on the hypogastric arteries as deep in the pelvis as possible (not shown).

The method for managing the distal end point when intimal thickening extends only into the first centimeter of the external iliac artery is illustrated in **Fig. 5.6a and b.** A transverse arteriotomy has been made in the common iliac artery just proximal to its bifurcation. The end of the atheroma in the external iliac artery is visible as a posterior tongue. The tip of a Beaver blade raises the atheroma to develop the distal end point. The dissection plane is then developed into the common iliac artery by insertion and spreading of the tips of a right-angle clamp (**Fig. 5.7a and b**). The object at this stage is to develop a core of freed intima around which an internal stripper can be passed (**Fig. 5.8**). Usually the stripper will remain in the original endarterectomy plane. Occasionally, when the atheroma involves only a portion of the iliac circumference, the stripper will leave the less diseased intima in place. After the stripper has been removed, palpation of the artery between the thumb and index finger may reveal portions of the arterial wall to be slightly thicker than adjacent portions. It is advisable to remove this remaining intimal layer either by repeated passages of the stripper or by instrumental extraction with a long angled hemostat. **Fig. 5.9a and b** are photographs of the arterial strippers we have designed for closed endarterectomy. The malleable silver handle allows the stripper to be shaped to accommodate to the restricted working area in the performance of a common iliac endarterectomy.

115

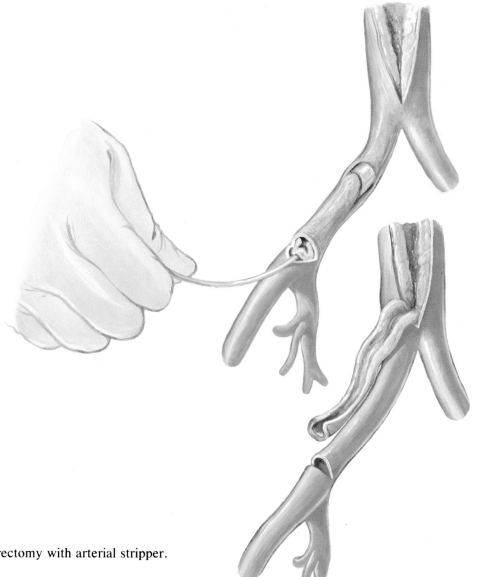

Fig. 5.8. Closed iliac endarterectomy with arterial stripper.

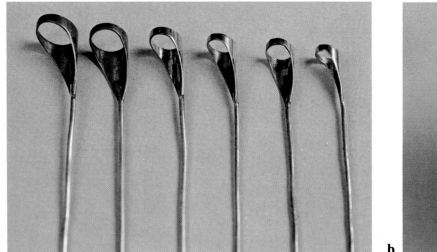

a

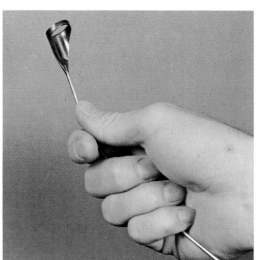

b

Fig. 5.9. **a** Intra-arterial strippers. The ferrule has an oblique and blunted leading edge and has been incorporated into the shaft for strength. **b** The malleable silver handle allows it to be bent for application in restricted areas. The stripper has its greatest usefulness for atherosclerosis in the common carotid, the common iliac, and occasionally the external iliac arteries.

When the external iliac lesion extends beyond the level where it can be reached through the common iliac arteriotomy, a transverse arteriotomy is made in the external iliac artery just beyond the palpable lesion. The posterior normal intima is incised and a proximal dissection plane is developed by gentle hoeing and cutting with the tip of the Beaver blade (**Fig. 5.10a**). The maneuver shown in Fig. 5.7a and b then creates a circumferential external iliac endarterectomy to the level of its orifice (**Fig. 5.10b**). The distal intima remains firmly attached and tack-down sutures are rarely necessary. **Fig. 5.11a and b** shows the completion of the aortic endarterectomy with transection of the intima at the level of the infrarenal clamp.

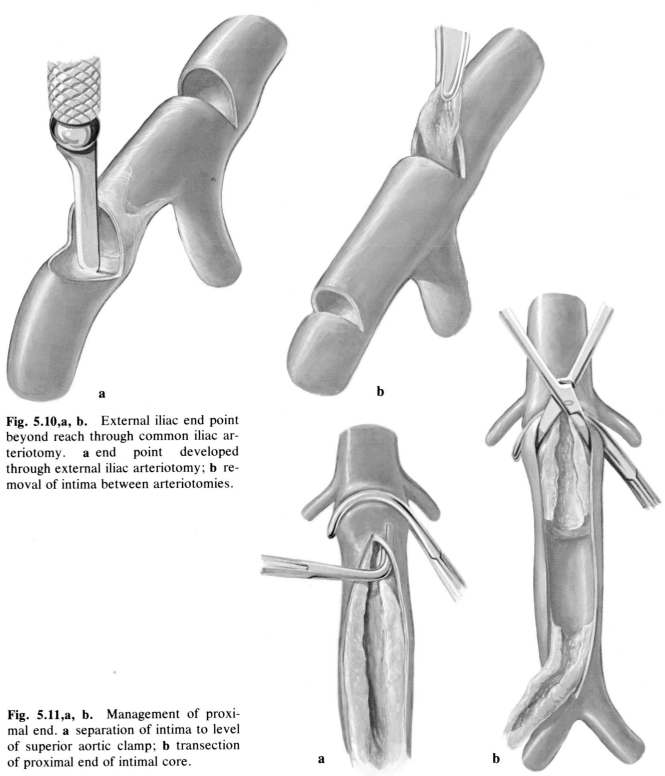

a

b

Fig. 5.10,a, b. External iliac end point beyond reach through common iliac arteriotomy. **a** end point developed through external iliac arteriotomy; **b** removal of intima between arteriotomies.

Fig. 5.11,a, b. Management of proximal end. **a** separation of intima to level of superior aortic clamp; **b** transection of proximal end of intimal core.

a

b

117

The final step in the operation is the removal of as much of the thickened hypogastric intima as is possible. Atherosclerosis rarely extends into the branches of the hypogastric artery. Although blind endarterectomy by instrumental extraction from a proximal arteriotomy is an unacceptable technique when the artery distal to the diseased segment can be exposed, it is the only technique that can be employed in this situation. With a finger behind the artery, the opened jaws of a hemostat can be guided along the dissection plane and the thickened intima extracted (**Fig. 5.12a and b**). After removal of the primary lesions, one can then remove any residual intimal fragments (**Fig. 5.12c**).

After completion of these maneuvers, the aorta is closed with a continuous 4–0 suture and the iliac arteriotomies are closed with interrupted 5–0 sutures.

In *type B distribution of atherosclerosis*, endarterectomy of the external iliac artery to and including the common femoral artery is feasible in most cases. The endarterectomy plane is first developed at the distal end through a longitudinal arteriotomy in the common femoral artery. An arterial stripper is then passed proximally into the external iliac artery, which should be done under direct vision with the artery stretched taut both proximal and distal to the stripper. Unless one does so, the artery will tend to buckle ahead of the stripper and allow it to penetrate the wall. The entry of the stripper into a plane deeper than desirable is revealed when the metallic hue of the stripper ring becomes visible. The most common place for this to occur is in the proximal portion of the external iliac artery. Removal of the stripper and substitution of one of a smaller size permits completion of the dissection without difficulty. After removal of the specimen, palpable differences in thickness of the arterial wall are often present due to the presence of residual undiseased intima. If the stripper can be passed through again without becoming entangled in redundant intima, this situation is usually benign and not conducive to thrombosis.

The alternate technique for endarterectomy of the external iliac artery is to remove the artery and use the eversion endarterectomy technique, following which the artery is returned to its original position with two anastomoses. The only disadvantage of this method is the necessity for dividing the inferior epigastric and circumflex iliac artery branches, the two arteries that provide a major source of collateral flow to the lower extremities in the event of postoperative or late iliac occlusion.

For most of our patients with type B aortoiliac atherosclerosis we have turned more and more to the bypass procedure for elective operations. A lengthy endarterectomy, which includes the external iliac arteries, performed by either of the methods described may be a limb-saving operation in patients with a previously placed bypass graft who have developed perigraft infection. We have managed these patients by removal of the graft and revascularization by autogenous tissue techniques.

Aortofemoral Bypass

For type B aortoiliac atherosclerosis, an aortobilateral common femoral bypass graft is the most commonly performed operation. As stated previously, the distribution of the atherosclerotic lesions includes the external iliac arteries and, usually to a lesser extent, the common femoral arteries as well. Although the superficial femoral arteries are usually involved to a varying degree, the ultimate objective of the operation is to provide normal inflow to the terminal branches of the profunda femoris arteries.

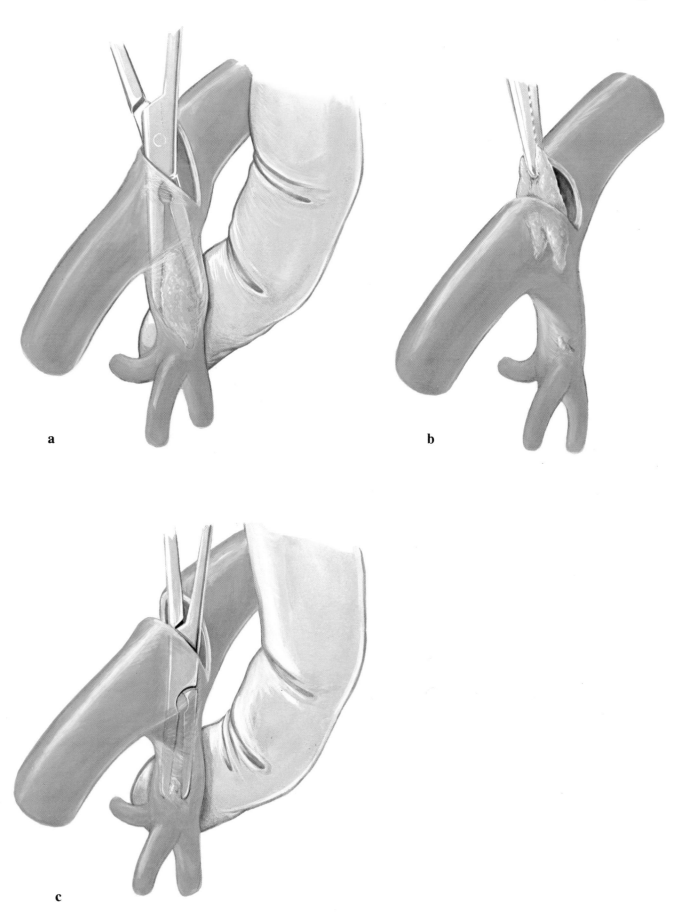

Fig. 5.12,a–c. Hypogastric endarterectomy. **a** development of intimal core with hemostat; **b** extraction of specimen (incomplete); **c** removal of residual fragments.

119

Disease in the external iliac arteries may be no more than a lengthy posterior plaque that may not be apparent on the preoperative aortogram. When this is the case, the abdomen is opened first to allow the surgeon to palpate the full length of the external iliac arteries through the intact posterior peritoneum before the decision is made to extend the operation to the groins. If the external iliac lesions are apparent on the aortogram, the groin dissections are completed first to lessen the time period of the abdominal portion of the operation.

Operative Technique

Incisions   The abdominal incision extends in the midline from the xiphoid to the symphysis pubis. Vertical groin incisions, centered at the inguinal ligament, are made over the common femoral arteries (**Fig. 5.13**). The distal end of these incisions should be extended to a level that provides exposure of the common femoral bifurcation to permit evaluation of the profunda orifices. As the incision is deepened (**Fig. 5.14**), inguinal nodes will usually be encountered and whenever possible should be preserved and retracted medially. This maneuver, as well as the strict avoidance of transverse or "hockey-stick" incision, lessens the risk of a subcutaneous lymph collection that may ultimately result in postoperative groin sepsis.

A 3-cm incision made across the anterior and posterior fibers of the inguinal ligament preserving the fibers of the external oblique muscle (**Fig. 5.15a**) permits the necessary exposure for transection and ligation of the circumflex iliac vein, which crosses the anterior surface of the external iliac artery 2–4 cm proximal to the shelving edge of the inguinal ligament (**Fig. 5.15b**). Disruption of this vein by blind finger dissection may produce bleeding that is difficult to control. Cutting the ligament also provides a larger tunnel for passage of the graft and avoids the occasional complication of graft compression at this site (**Fig. 5.16**). Postoperative femoral hernia requiring repair has not occurred.

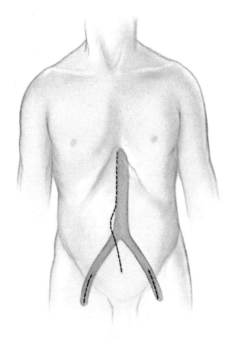

Fig. 5.13.   Full-length longitudinal midline incision.

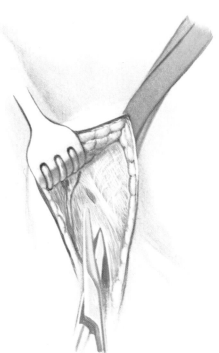

Fig. 5.14.   Groin incision centered over inguinal ligaments.

120

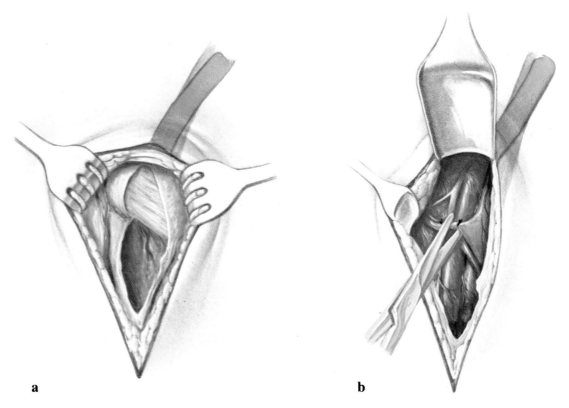

a   b

Fig. 5.15,a, b. Development of groin exposure. **a** transection of anterior and posterior fibers of inguinal ligament; **b** division of circumflex iliac vein.

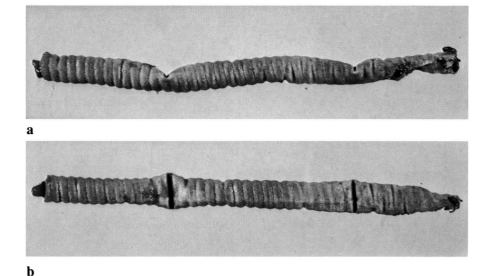

a

b

Fig. 5.16,a, b. Operative photograph of a chronically occluded iliac limb of an aortofemoral graft. The compression defect in the graft, which was thought to be the cause of occlusion, was at the point where it passed behind the inguinal ligament. Routine transection of the lower fibers of the ligament at the initial operation simplifies the procedure and preserves an adequate tunnel through which the graft can pass.

Preparation for Positioning of Graft   In **Fig. 5.17a** the posterior peritoneum over the aorta has been incised and a tunnel to the right groin incision is being developed. The dissecting finger inserted along the surface of the iliac arteries and posterior to the ureter will pass through an avascular plane with minimal resistance. A graft placed behind the ureter does not cause ureteral obstruction if it is placed without excessive tension.

A long clamp is passed from the groin to the end of the left index finger (**Fig. 5.17b**), and with the finger as a guide is advanced into the abdominal cavity (**Fig. 5.17c**). A rubber tube is then drawn through the tunnel to provide a guide for the later passage of the graft (**Fig. 5.17d**). On the left side, it is safer to develop this tunnel in two stages (using a retroperitoneal incision in the left iliac fossa) and to develop it also posterior to the ureter to lessen the chance for disruption of vessels at the base of the sigmoid mesentery. When an end-to-side proximal aorta–graft anastomosis is used, the tunnel also follows the course of the arteries; when the proximal anastomosis is end-to-end, the tunnel is developed in a more lateral position to be described later.

The tunnels are prepared in advance in order to lessen the period of ischemia when the aorta is clamped later in the operation. In addition, the preliminary retroperitoneal dissection lessens the troublesome bleeding

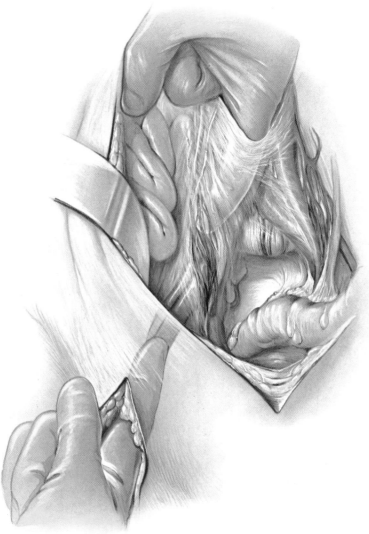

Fig. 5.17a

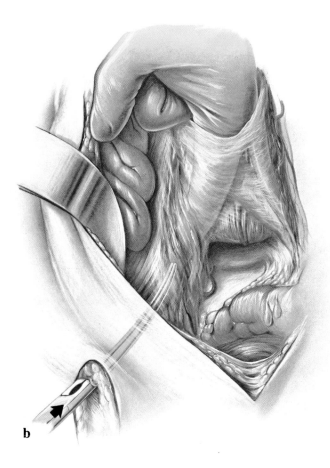

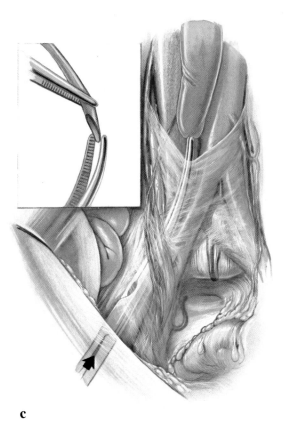

b

c

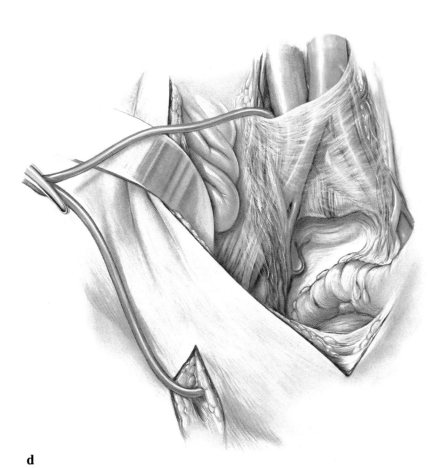

d

Fig. 5.17, a–d. Preparation of retro-peritoneal tunnel. **a** finger dissection along course of iliac artery; **b** introduction of clamp; **c** clamp replaced by latex tubing; **d** tubing in place as guide for passage of graft.

123

Aortoiliac Atherosclerosis

that may occur if the tunnels are created at a time when systemic heparinization has been induced.

Graft Size   The graft size should be related to the capacity of the efferent vessels. When the blood flow from the graft supplies patent superficial femoral and profunda femoris arteries as well as retrograde flow into patent external iliac arteries, the maximum graft size in the average male patient should not exceed 16 × 8 mm. We have found a 14 × 7 mm graft to be more appropriate in at least one-half of the male patients. (The arterial diameters of the distal arteries in women are smaller, and the graft size is reduced proportionately.) When the only distal patent efferent artery is the profunda femoris, either a 12 × 6 mm or a 10 × 5 mm graft provides iliac conduits of appropriate size. Oversized grafts reduce flow velocity in the graft and laminar flow contributes to circumferential mural thrombus in the wall of the graft, both of which are conducive to early or late graft occlusion. Many surgeons have been reluctant to use lengthy 5 or 6 mm graft segments for fear that the small diameter will contribute to occlusion. Although this may be a factor in low-flow situations (i.e., a femoropopliteal graft with distal disease), we have never encountered a problem with graft thrombosis from the use of a smaller graft when the outflow tract (superficial femoral and/or profunda) supplies the entire limb.

End-to-Side Proximal Anastomosis   The technique originally favored for establishing the aortic end of the graft is to anastomose it to the anterior surface of the aorta. It is a method which we only rarely use at this time. A longitudinal aortotomy of appropriate length **(Fig. 5.18)** is made in the segment of the aorta between the renal arteries and the inferior mesenteric artery (IMA). Loose debris within the aortic lumen is freed by vigorous flushing. A supplementary endarterectomy in this segment is generally not advised because of the difficulty in creating an adequate distal end point in the usually friable and degenerated intima. The anterior bulge of the aortic portion of the prosthesis will more than compensate for subsequent further thickening of the aortic wall. The aortic portion of the graft is transected as closely as possible to its bifurcation. The cephalad origin of the iliac limbs allows each to assume a more gentle curve as they deviate away from the midline than if the graft bifurcation had been placed at the anatomic level of the aortic bifurcation. The graft is sutured to the aorta using a running 3–0 or 4–0 synthetic suture.

After completion of the anastomosis, the aorta is flushed by alternate release of the proximal and distal clamps **(Fig. 5.19a and b)**. The aortic flow is then released into the hypogastric arteries for several minutes to flush away any residual aortic fragments into the pelvic circulation **(Fig. 5.19c)**.

Two major complications may result from the end-to-side technique just described. One is embolization to distal arteries. It is often difficult to remove all of the shaggy material within the aortic lumen at the site of the anastomosis. In addition, the intima within the jaws of the distal aortic clamp is susceptible to fragmentation and despite all of the flushing maneuvers is still vulnerable to late separation. Second, the aortic portion of the graft bulges anteriorly against the posterior surface of the duodenum, and the interposition of tissue between the two may be difficult to accomplish. Unopposed contact between a fabric graft and any segment of the intestine predisposes to erosion of the intestinal wall, aortoenteric fistulization, and perigraft sepsis. Even when tissue is placed between the graft and the duodenum it is likely to be vulnerable to erosion by compression from the forward bulge of the graft.

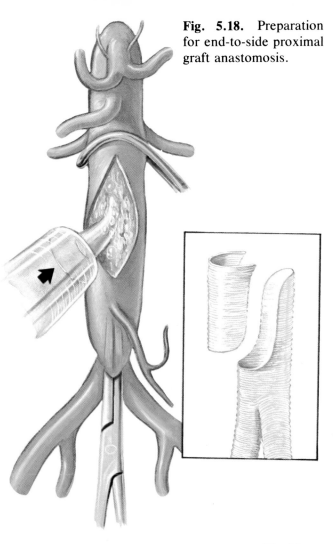

Fig. 5.18. Preparation for end-to-side proximal graft anastomosis.

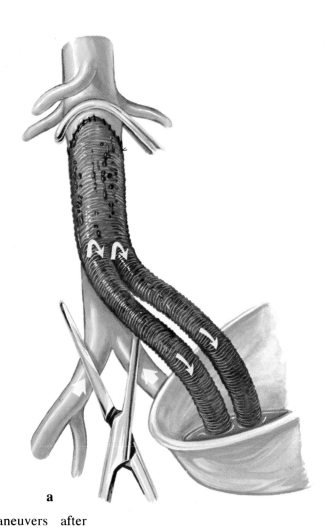

a

Fig. 5.19,a–c. Flushing maneuvers after completion of proximal anastomosis. **a** retrograde into graft; **b** antegrade into graft; **c** antegrade into hypogastric arteries.

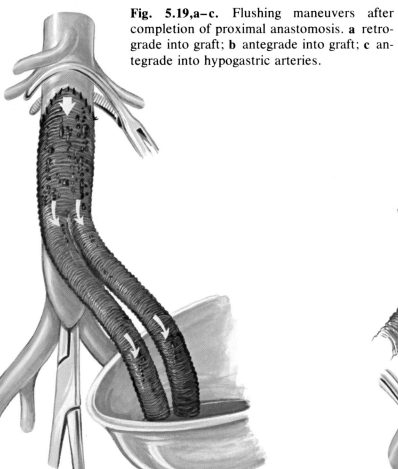

b

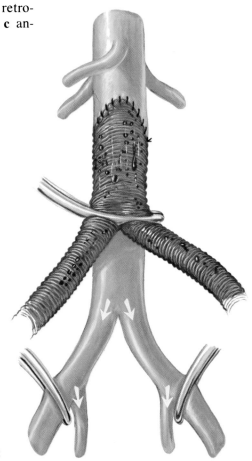

c

125

End-to-End Proximal Anastomosis   An alternate and now the preferable technique is to establish an end-to-end anastomosis to the transected infrarenal aorta. The short aortic portion of the graft lies in a normal posterior position and does not bulge forward against the duodenum. The right iliac arm of the graft lies between the aorta and the cava and usually can be positioned to protrude forward to cross the cava caudad to the duodenum. There are two theoretical disadvantages of this technique. Should perigraft sepsis develop, the graft could not be simply removed and the aorta reconstructed as with an end-to-side technique. Some form of a remote subcutaneous bypass graft would, therefore, be required to maintain extremity flow after removal of the graft. The other disadvantage is the potential for visceral ischemia by the reduction of forward flow from the aorta into any distal branches that may remain patent. Our own frequency of perigraft sepsis with end-to-end grafts (for aneurysm or aortofemoral bypass operations) has been less than 0.2%, and we have encountered only two complications of visceral ischemia from the use of a proximal end-to-end anastomosis for both aneurysmal or occlusive disease in the last 18 years. On the basis of this experience the disadvantage of this technique is more theoretical than real. In addition, the use of the end-to-end technique for aortofemoral bypass operations has eliminated the previously rare although occasionally disastrous complication of distal embolization.

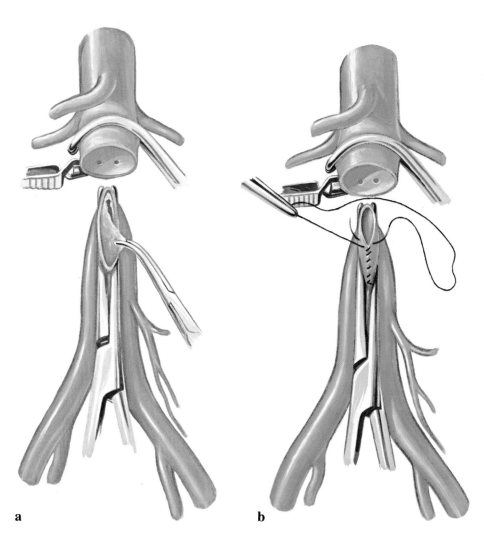

Fig. 5.20,a, b. Preparation for end-to-end proximal graft anastomosis. **a** intima extracted from distal aortic stump after resection of short segment of aorta; **b** closure of distal aortic stump.

a   b

126

Fig. 5.20a illustrates the first step in preparing the aorta for this anastomosis. Aortic clamps have been applied across the infrarenal aorta and obliquely across the aorta proximal to the IMA. A 4-cm segment of the aorta between the clamps is resected. If there is substantial thickening of the aortic wall in the proximal stump, the intima in this segment is extracted. The intima in the distal stump proximal to the clamp is extracted to permit a tight closure (**Fig. 5.20b**). The aortic portion of the graft is transected to leave a 4-cm aortic shaft for anastomosis.

One technical maneuver not illustrated in the drawings is critically important. The back flow from the inferior mesenteric and lumbar arteries may be sufficient to maintain forward flow through the occluded distal aortic stump until the distal graft limb anastomoses have become operational. If the operation is being performed to bypass stenotic lesions in the aorta or iliac arteries, embolization to the legs can occur at this time from fragments of crushed intima dislodged by the application of the distal aortic clamp. This complication can be prevented by occluding the external iliac arteries until forward flow through the iliac graft limbs has been created.

When the end-to-end technique is used, there is one difference in the method of routing the left iliac arm of the graft. The retroperitoneal incision lateral to the sigmoid mesentery is extended to a more proximal level. A dissection plane is then developed on the anterior surface of the psoas muscle to a level cephalad to the origin of the IMA. With finger dissection one can then tunnel to the left side of the aorta with less risk of damaging the vessels in the left colon mesentery than if a lower approach were to be used. The left iliac arm of the graft brought through this tunnel immediately occupies a position posterior to the branches of the IMA and the ureter and is completely shielded from contact with the duodenum. This, of course, can only be accomplished if the aortic shaft is short, as described.

The graft is sutured to the aortic stump with slight clockwise rotation of the graft to allow the right iliac limb to cross the inferior vena cava distal to the duodenum without kinking at its origin and the left iliac limb to drop into a position on to the anterior surface of the left psoas muscle and posterior to the vessels in the sigmoid mesentery (**Fig. 5.21**). The only portion of the graft that projects forward into the abdomen beyond the anterior surface of the aorta is the right iliac limb, and this is easily covered by suturing the peritoneum on the left to the retroduodenal soft tissue. **Figs. 5.22 and 5.23a and b** are photographs from two operations illustrating the proximal anastomosis and the ease with which the graft is covered.

127

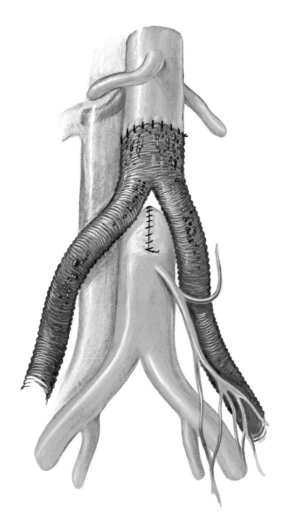

Fig. 5.21. Route of iliac limbs of the graft with end-to-end proximal anastomosis.

Fig. 5.22. Proximal end of an aorta–bifemoral bypass graft in a patient with degenerative intimal disease adjacent to the level of the renal arteries. A suprarenal clamp was used to permit a level for anastomosis adjacent to the renal arteries. The origin of the right renal artery can be seen in the left lower corner. A segment of the aorta has been resected to provide a posterior position for the aortic portion of the graft. In situations such as this it is advisable to clamp the IMA as well as the external iliac arteries until the distal anastomoses have been completed.

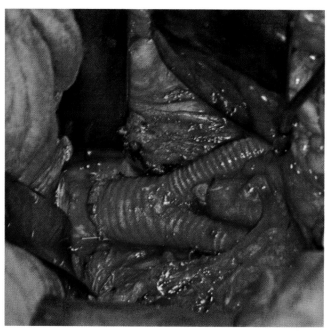

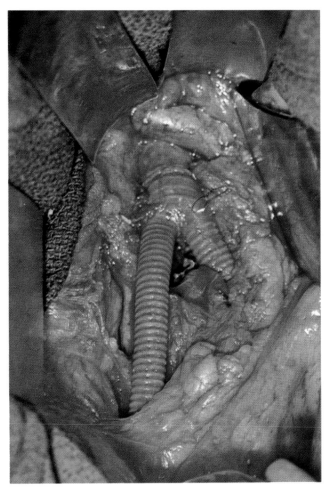

a

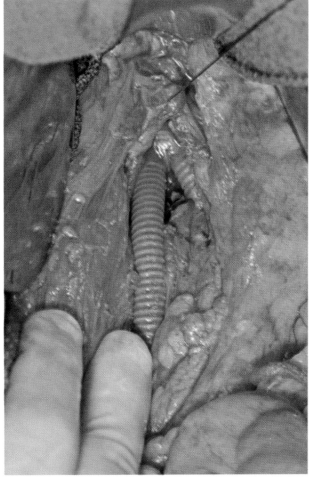

b

Fig. 5.23,a, b. Retroperitoneal isolation of bypass graft. **a** An infrarenal aorta–bifemoral bypass graft has been placed with an end-to-end proximal anastomosis. The left iliac arm of the graft extends posterior to the vascular arcade of the branches of the inferior mesenteric artery. The most anterior position of the graft is that of the right iliac arm as it passes in front of the inferior vena cava. Note the ridge of soft tissue that has been preserved on each side of the original position of the aorta. **b** Beginning approximation of the retroperitoneal soft tissue to cover the graft and isolate it from contact with the duodenum.

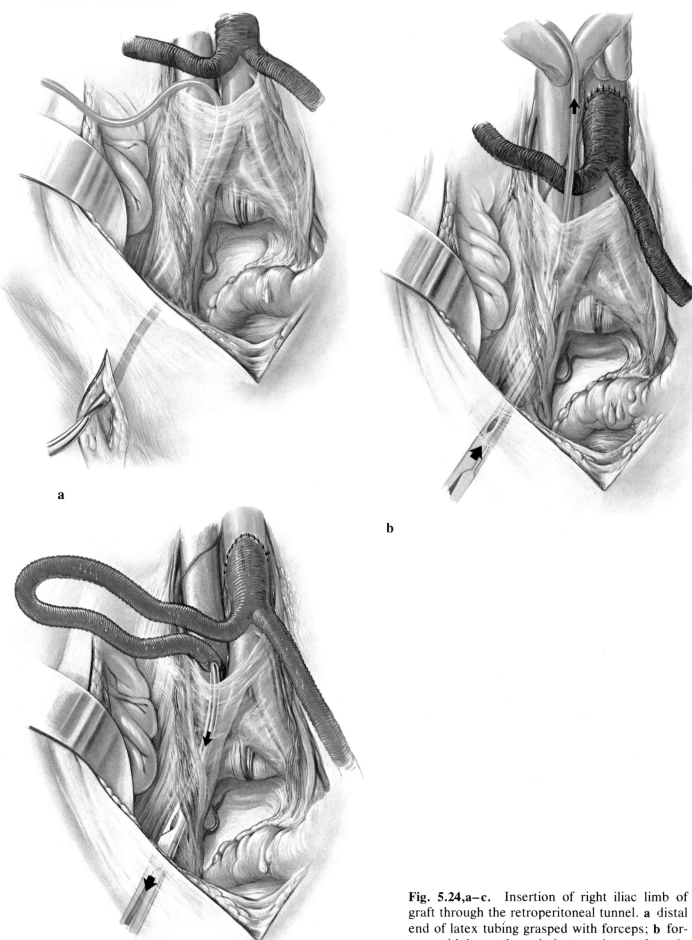

Fig. 5.24, a–c. Insertion of right iliac limb of graft through the retroperitoneal tunnel. **a** distal end of latex tubing grasped with forceps; **b** forceps withdrawn through the tunnel; **c** graft ready for introduction into the preformed tunnel.

a

b

c

Femoral Anastomosis The maneuvers for reintroduction of the clamp that is to be used for pulling the iliac arms of the graft into the groin incisions are shown in **Fig. 5.24a–c.** In these illustrations an end-to-side proximal anastomosis has been established to the aorta.

Before the decision is made to terminate the operation with end-to-side graft to the anterior surface of the common femoral artery, careful assessment of the degree and extent of atherosclerosis in the common femoral and profunda femoris arteries must be made. Although disease in these segments does not interfere with the successful completion of the anastomosis, later progression of disease may result in graft occlusion. Preliminary assessment of the extent of disease is aided by the preoperative arteriogram, but the definitive evaluation occurs at the operating table. The arterial segment is palpated and after the common femoral arteriotomy has been made the interior of the common femoral artery and the orifices of the outflow arteries are inspected.

In the type B aortoiliac disease for which an aortofemoral graft is being used, some degree of atherosclerosis in the common femoral artery is usually encountered. In its simplest form, mild thickening of the posterior wall tapers off to a normal intima proximal to the orifice of the profunda femoris. In this situation, the distal profunda femoris remains free of disease. The broad surface of the spatulated end of a graft anastomosed to the side of the common femoral artery opposite the atheroma makes it unlikely that progression of the atheroma will compromise the lumen at this level. The femoral arteriotomy should be placed in the center of the uninvolved portion of the circumference of the artery. This thin and easily indented portion is usually on the anterior surface of the artery but occasionally may be located on one side or the other.

Often the atheroma will extend distally into one side of the profunda orifice. This can usually be determined by palpation of the proximal profunda with a curved hemostat behind it (**Fig. 5.25**). If the lesion is small and does not surround the profunda orifice, the common femoral arteriotomy may be extended into the profunda opposite the lesion and the graft extended onto the profunda as a patch.

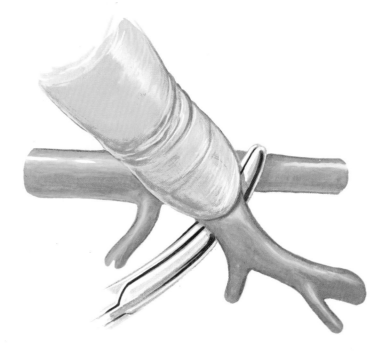

Fig. 5.25. Palpation of the profunda orifice.

131

More advanced lesions in the common femoral artery tend to involve more of its circumference, narrow its lumen appreciably, and extend into the full circumference of the profunda orifice. The intima of the superficial femoral artery, if patent, will usually be thickened in varying degrees along its course. The simple techniques described above will provide a satisfactory immediate result but invite late graft occlusion as the lesions progress. A more complete and durable reconstruction requires endarterectomy of the common femoral artery with extension into the profunda femoris and superficial femoral arteries.

If the profunda lesion involves only its orifice, the thickened intima may often be safely removed through the common femoral arteriotomy. If the profunda lesion is more lengthy (and the superficial femoral artery is patent), a profunda angioplasty to the distal level of palpable or visible disease is required. The description of various techniques for this operation is supplied in Volume II under "Femoropopliteal Reconstruction."

A technique that has been useful in gauging the appropriate tension of the iliac arms of the graft is illustrated in Fig. 5.26a–d. With the graft pulled taut, it is cut 5 cm longer than would seem proper (**Fig. 5.26a**). After the femoral anastomosis is completed using running 5–0 or 6–0 synthetic sutures, flow is first opened into the proximal iliac artery (**Fig. 5.26b**). The clamp on a patent superficial femoral artery is the last part to be removed, thus avoiding possible embolization to the distal leg or foot. After release

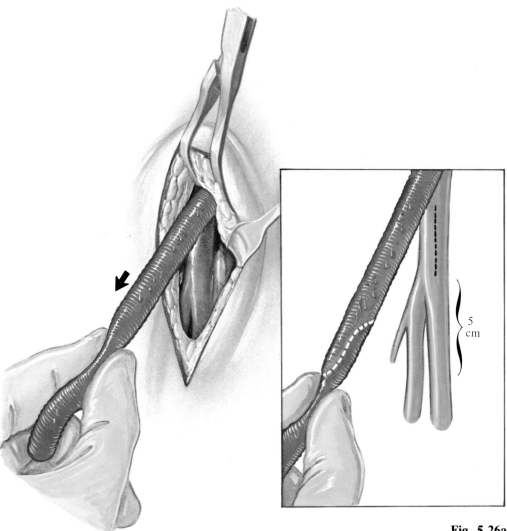

5 cm

Fig. 5.26a

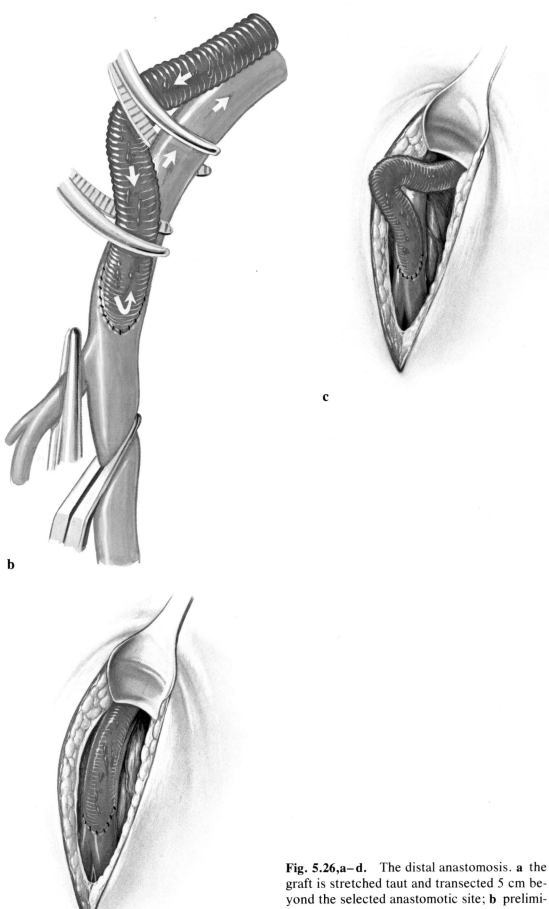

c

b

d

Fig. 5.26,a–d. The distal anastomosis. **a** the graft is stretched taut and transected 5 cm beyond the selected anastomotic site; **b** preliminary retrograde flush of graft; **c** redundant distal graft; **d** graft withdrawn into abdomen.

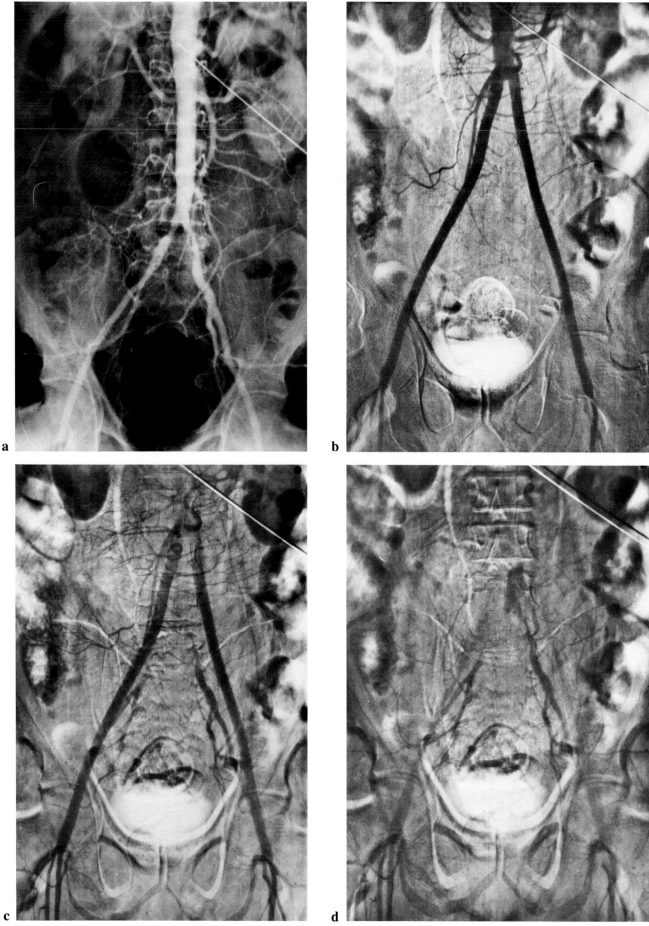

a

b

c

d

Fig. 5.27

of the remaining clamps the redundant portion of the graft is withdrawn into the abdominal cavity (**Fig. 5.26c and d**). This releases the tension in the iliac portion of the graft and the inflow segment into the femoral artery assumes an appropriate contour. The arteriographic appearance of a functioning aortofemoral graft is shown in **Fig. 5.27a–d.**

Infrarenal Aortic Occlusion

Atherosclerotic occlusion of the infrarenal abdominal aorta that has progressed upward to a level subjacent to the renal artery orifices is a pattern of disease requiring special consideration. The significant feature of this lesion is the intraluminal thrombus at its cephalad end. The primary occluding atherosclerotic lesion is often confined to the distal half to two-thirds of the infrarenal aorta or even the iliac arteries. With the onset of distal occlusion, the aortic outflow becomes confined to the inferior mesenteric and lumbar arteries, and the lumen of the patent infrarenal aortic segment becomes progressively narrowed by a layer of mural thrombus that often extends upward to within a centimeter of the renal arteries. When performing endarterectomy or bypass operations for distal aortic occlusion, the surgeon must be aware of the probability of proximal mural thrombosis and should place the proximal aortic clamp as closely subjacent as possible to, or even above, the renal arteries.

When the mural thrombus in the infrarenal aorta progresses to occlusion, the cephalad propagation of thrombus extends to the level of the renal arteries where it is arrested, at least temporarily, by the rapid outflow of blood into the renal arteries. Continuing buildup of thrombus eventually leads to occlusion of the renal arteries and, in some patients, even of the superior mesenteric artery. Although the usual symptom of subrenal aorta occlusion is only simple claudication, the potential for a lethal complication presents a stronger indication for operation than is present in other distributions of aortoiliac atherosclerosis.

The selection of bypass grafting or endarterectomy or a combination of the two is based upon conditions previously discussed in this chapter. Both operations are equally satisfactory for dealing with the aortic portion of the disease. With either method particular attention is paid to the prevention of thrombotic embolization to the renal arteries. Both require gen-

Fig. 5.27,a–d. Preoperative (**a**) and postoperative (**b, c, d**) aortograms in a patient with atherosclerotic aortoiliac stenosis treated by an aortofemoral bypass graft. The preoperative aortogram suggests that disease is localized to the region of the aortic bifurcation. At laparotomy, posterior intimal thickening was palpated in the full length of both external iliac arteries. There was no palpable disease in the aorta proximal to the IMA.

A 14 × 7-mm Dacron bifurcation graft was anastomosed end-to-end to the infrarenal aorta and the iliac arms of the graft were extended to the sides of the common femoral arteries bilaterally. Note the lateral position of the left iliac arm, which passes behind the IMA and the vascular arcade in the left mesocolon to course along the surface of the left psoas muscle. Retrograde flow in the external iliac arteries (**d**) provides blood flow to the pelvic vessels. This route of pelvic flow can be considered no more than temporary since it will be lost once the iliac arteries become occluded by atherosclerosis. As long as the superior mesenteric artery remains patent, adequate collateral flow can be anticipated from that source.

135

tle mobilization of the infrarenal abdominal aorta and temporary clamping of the suprarenal aorta and the renal arteries (**Fig. 5.28a**).

If a bypass graft is to be used, we prefer using an end-to-end proximal anastomosis. The aorta is transected at a level that will permit inspection of the renal orifices after the thrombus has been removed. The thrombus is gently extracted piecemeal from the proximal stump (**Fig. 5.28b**). Thickening of the intima is usually minimal. Care should be employed to prevent disrupting the intima. After the anastomosis has been completed (**Fig. 5.28c**), the aorta is flushed by temporary release of the aortic clamps while the renal artery clamps are still in place. The aortic clamp is then transferred to an infrarenal position and blood flow restored to the renal arteries while the distal portion of the operation is completed. Renal ischemia time rarely exceeds 15–20 min.

An alternate technique is illustrated in **Fig. 5.29a–c**. Thrombus has partially obstructed the right renal orifice and certain total extraction from below may be difficult to accomplish. The thrombus is extracted through a longitudinal aortotomy placed between the renal arteries to permit more direct inspection of the renal orifices after the thrombus has been removed. For purposes of exposition, an additional, but not necessarily associated,

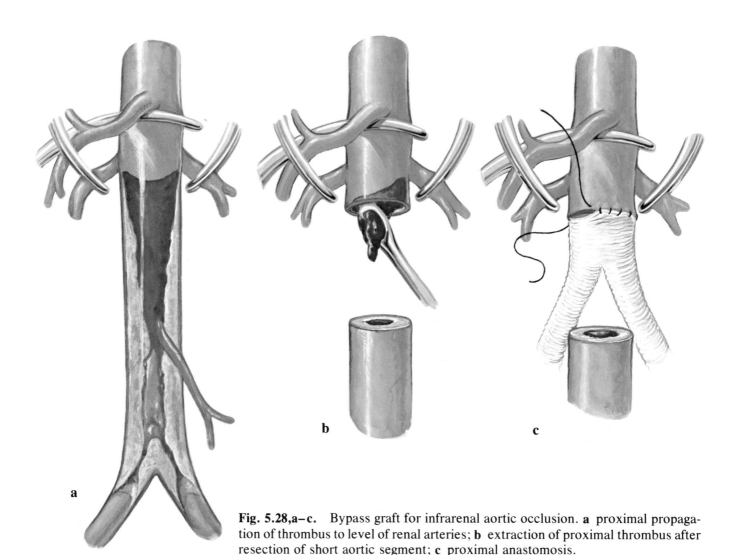

Fig. 5.28, a–c. Bypass graft for infrarenal aortic occlusion. **a** proximal propagation of thrombus to level of renal arteries; **b** extraction of proximal thrombus after resection of short aortic segment; **c** proximal anastomosis.

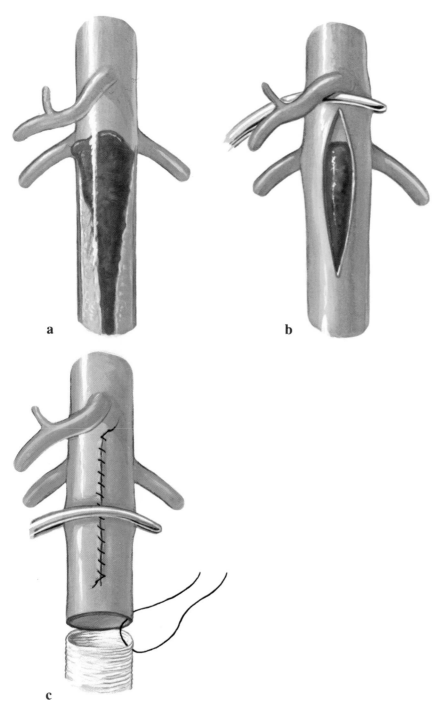

a

b

c

Fig. 5.29,a–c. Bypass graft combined with proximal endarterectomy (for infrarenal aortic occlusion). **a** extensive atherosclerosis and pararenal extension of thrombus; **b** longitudinal aortotomy extending proximal to renal orifices; **c** proximal thrombectomy and endarterectomy completed and aorta prepared for graft anastomosis.

pathologic variant has been introduced, i.e., extensive atherosclerotic intimal disease approaching the level of the renal arteries. In this situation the intima in the infrarenal segment should be removed by endarterectomy before the graft is anastomosed. When preparing the aorta for the graft anastomosis it is helpful to preserve a small endarterectomized aortic cuff between the distal end of the aortotomy and the point of transection (**Fig. 5.29c**).

137

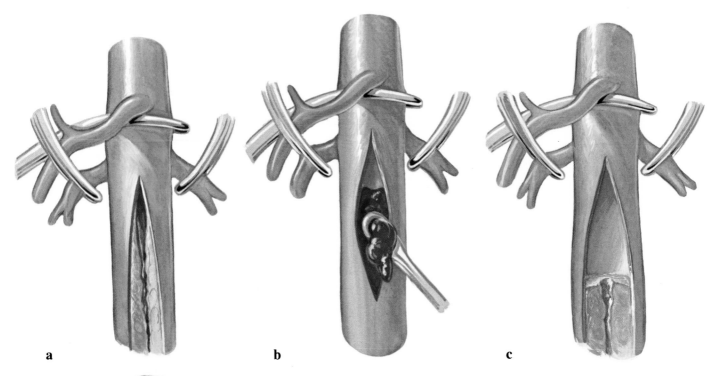

a   b   c

Fig. 5.30,a–d. Endarterectomy for infrarenal aortic occlusion. **a** aortotomy in occluded aorta; **b** removal of proximal thrombus; **c** endarterectomized proximal aorta; **d** renal flow restored before completion of endarterectomy.

d

When endarterectomy is selected as the definitive operation for the aortoiliac disease, the steps in its performance at the renal level are those shown in **Fig. 5.30a–d**. The customary longitudinal aortotomy is extended proximally to a level at the upper edge of the thrombus. The intima in the first 4–5 cm of the infrarenal aorta is removed to permit closure of the aortotomy and transfer of the aortic clamp before completing the rest of the aortoiliac endarterectomy.

Crossover Grafts

"Crossover" grafts from one external iliac or common femoral artery to the contralateral common femoral or profunda femoris artery for the management of unilateral iliac obstructive disease is an alternate technique (**Fig. 5.31**) to the more direct techniques described previously. It is applicable only when there is normal blood flow on the donor side, when aortography demonstrates a widely patent lumen in the afferent portions of the parent artery, and when it is unlikely that progression of atherosclerosis

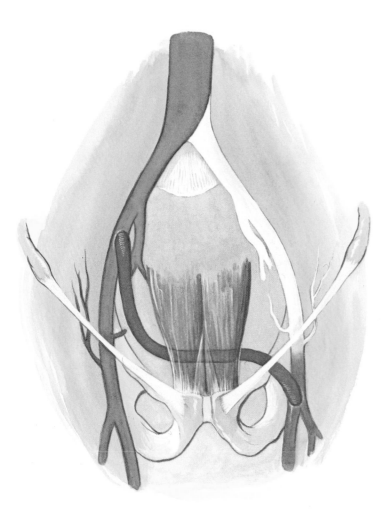

Fig. 5.31. Iliac–femoral crossover graft.

will lead to reduction of blood flow in the parent artery during the patient's anticipated life span. Its use is consequently largely restricted to elderly patients in whom, for various reasons excluding that of age alone, it would be inadvisable to perform a direct and more durable intra-abdominal operation. These include patients who have undergone previous transperitoneal but unsuccessful revascularization operations, patients who have had peritonitis or numerous laparotomies, and patients who have a minimal respiratory reserve. The operation is usually used only in patients with findings or symptoms of severe ischemia.

Only rarely will the outflow tract require a graft larger than 6 mm in diameter. The proximal end of the graft is anastomosed to the donor external iliac artery at the junction of its middle and distal thirds. Access to this segment is obtained through either a vertical groin incision in which the inguinal ligament is partially transected or, preferably, through an oblique lower-quadrant abdominal incision with a retroperitoneal approach. Anastomosis to the external iliac artery at this level allows minimum deviation of flow direction in the first portion of the graft and the creation of a gentle curve in the graft as it turns to cross the lower abdominal wall just cephalad to the symphysis pubis. The previously described technique of preparing one limb of a graft from a bifurcation graft is often useful in this situation. A less desirable situation occurs when the femoral artery is used as the donor site; the graft is obliged to angle in a retrograde direction to enter the suprapubic transabdominal tunnel.

The transabdominal tunnel is placed behind the rectus muscles through the space of Retzius, a plane easily developed with finger dissection. A graft in this position is not subject to compression when the patient is lying in the prone position, as would a graft in the subcutaneous level. Partial transection of the inguinal ligament adjacent to the pubis on the recipient side allows the graft to exit without compression and at a level proximal to the femoral artery on the recipient side. If the graft is cut to be slightly longer than necessary, it will assume another gentle curve as it falls into position paralleling the femoral artery. **Fig. 5.32** shows the arteriographic appearance of a functioning iliac–femoral crossover graft.

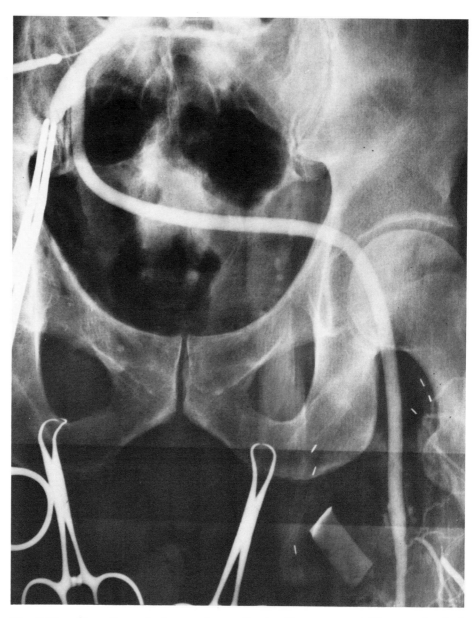

Fig. 5.32. Operative arteriogram in a patient with an external iliac–profunda femoris crossover graft. This patient had undergone three previous transabdominal attempts at aortofemoral reconstruction, all of which had undergone late failure. The left iliac arm of the most recent aorta–bifemoral graft has occluded acutely. The left superficial femoral artery is thrombosed. A 6-mm PTFE graft has been anastomosed to the side of the patent right iliac arm of the previous graft and extended across the abdomen in the space of Retzius and anastomosed end-to-end to the left profunda femoris artery.

The following case histories, photographs, and aortograms (**Figs. 5.33–5.47**) illustrate the implications of the natural history and pathologic variations of aortoiliac atherosclerotic occlusive disease on various aspects of surgical management.

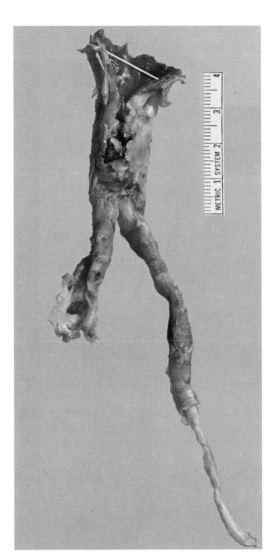

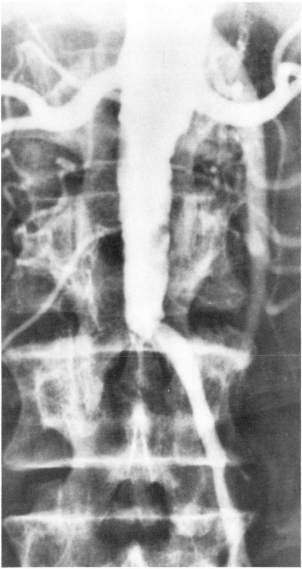

Fig. 5.33. Endarterectomy specimen in a patient with occlusive atherosclerosis of the terminal abdominal aorta and common iliac arteries, in whom the infrarenal aorta and both external iliac arteries were patent. Note the atherosclerotic thickening that has already developed in the wall of the proximal patent half of the infrarenal aorta and the circumferential mural thrombus which has appeared in response to restriction of aortic outflow. In the iliac segments, the disease has extended on one side into the first centimeter of the external iliac artery. In the other side, a lengthy tongue of an external iliac atheroma involves the proximal two-thirds of the artery. This is the distribution of disease that nowadays would indicate a reconstructive operation to the level of the common femoral arteries, usually by means of a bypass graft.

Fig. 5.34. Aortogram of a patient with atherosclerotic occlusion of the distal aorta. Thrombotic occlusion has progressed proximally to the origin of the IMA. Thrombus partially encircling the origin of the IMA is visible. An intraluminal shell of thrombus has ascended to the level of the renal arteries. In the natural progression of this lesion, one can anticipate gradual occlusion of the IMA by thrombus and subsequent thrombotic occlusion of the aorta to the level of the renal arteries. At operation, it becomes necessary to mobilize the infrarenal aorta with extreme care and to apply the aortic clamp proximal to the renal arteries. Endarterectomy of the infrarenal aorta to a point just distal to the IMA was performed. The aorta was transected as that point, and to its end was anastomosed a 14 × 7 mm bifurcation graft; the iliac graft limbs were anastomosed to the common femoral arteries.

141

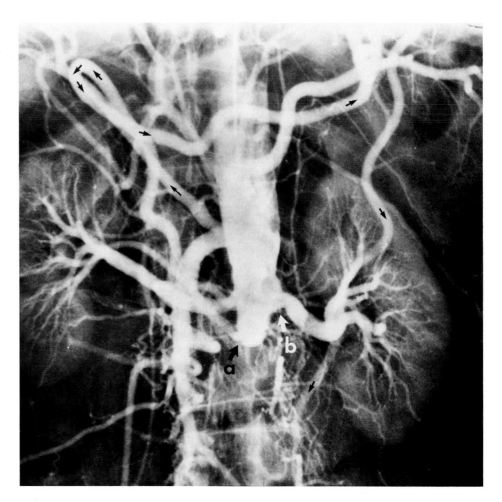

Fig. 5.35. Catheter aortogram (transaxillary route) in a patient with atherosclerotic infrarenal aortic occlusion. The proximal level of occlusion is at the caudad edge of the orifice of the distal of two renal arteries to the right kidney (*a*). Mural thrombus has propogated along the left lateral wall of the aorta to the level of and slightly into the orifice of the left renal artery (*b*). The contribution of the left colic branch of the SMA to collateral blood supply to the left colon is demonstrated (serial arrows). At operation the proximal aortic clamp should be placed either proximal to the celiac artery or just distal to the SMA. Mobilization of the aorta at the supraceliac level lessens the hazard of dislodging mural thrombus and embolization into the renal arteries.

Fig. 5.36,a, b. Preoperative (**a**) aortogram in a 56-year-old female with atherosclerotic occlusion of the infrarenal aorta with proximal progression of thrombus that almost occludes a low right renal artery (*a*) and narrows the aorta to the level of the SMA (*b*) and the left renal artery (*c*). Note the left colic branch of the SMA (*d*), which has become a portion of the collateral supply to the left colon. **b** Postoperative aortogram.

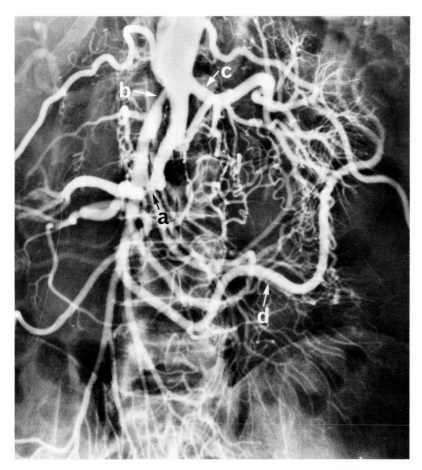

Fig. 5.36a

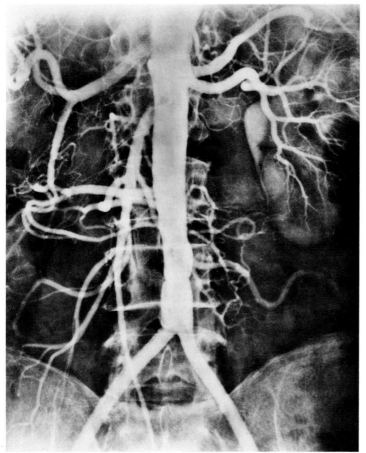

Fig. 5.36b

143

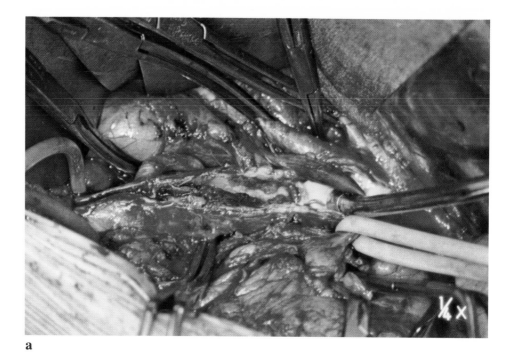

a

Fig. 5.37,a–g. Successive steps in the operation performed upon the patient whose aortograms are shown in Figs. 5.36a and b. A thoracoretroperitoneal abdominal approach has been used to expose the full length of the abdominal aorta and the iliac arteries with supplemental incisions in the groins to expose the common femoral arteries. **a** A longitudinal aortotomy has been made from the celiac artery (clamped superiorly at the far right) to beyond the origin of the left renal artery (lifted superiorly with a curved clamp at the far left). Latex tubing and a sucker provide cephalad retraction of the left renal vein. The clamp to the lower left is on an accessory left renal artery, which later was found to be totally occluded. The left renal artery is occluded by a clamp, the tip of which is out of view behind the left renal vein. The anterior wall of the aorta at the level of the superior mesenteric artery (occluded with a clamp above the left renal vein) shows moderate atherosclerotic thickening. The most obvious pathologic abnormality is intraluminal thrombus in the aorta. It totally occludes the segment distal to the right renal artery and extends cephalad to surround the orifice of the right renal artery and further to cover the right lateral surface of the aorta to within a cm of the orifice of the superior mesenteric artery. Introduction of the tip of a right-angle clamp showed a lumen of normal size in the orifices of both the SMA and the left renal artery. **b** A preliminary attempt at simple thrombectomy uncovered a thick ledge of aortic atheroma to which the thrombus had become attached. Atheromatous thickening at the orifice of the right renal artery was also palpable. **c** Aortic endarterectomy was started at the cephalad end of gross disease, caudad to the SMA orifice and sparing the intima at the orifice of the left renal artery. **d** Endarterectomy at the orifice of the accessory left renal artery failed to reach an end point in this artery. **e** A cylinder of aortic intima including the orifice lesion in the right renal artery has been dissected free. **f** The endarterectomy specimen is transected when the dissection has progressed to a level where the aortotomy may be closed and renal blood flow restored. Note the orifice of the right renal artery in the center of the exposure. **g** The aortotomy has been closed after a renal ischemia time of 20 min. The operation is concluded with a 12 × 6-mm bifurcation graft anastomosed end-to-end to the endarterectomized aortic stump and end-to-side to the common femoral arteries.

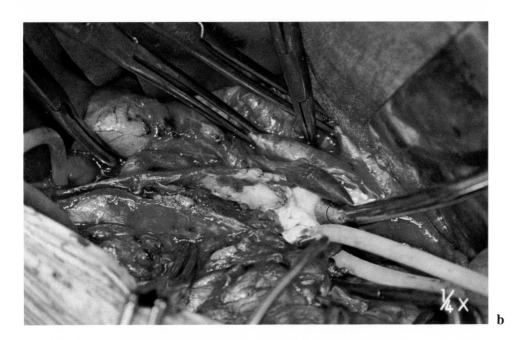

b

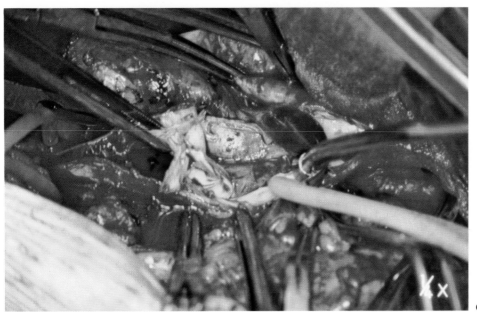

c

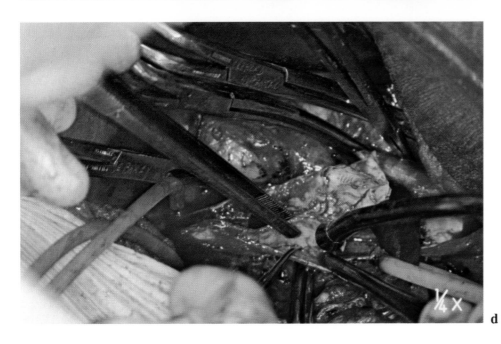

d   **Fig. 5.37** (cont.)

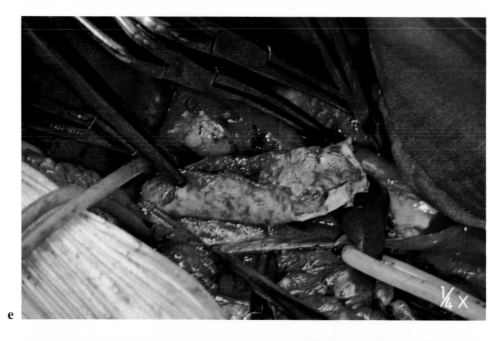

e

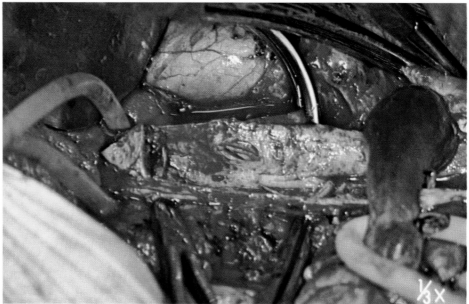

f

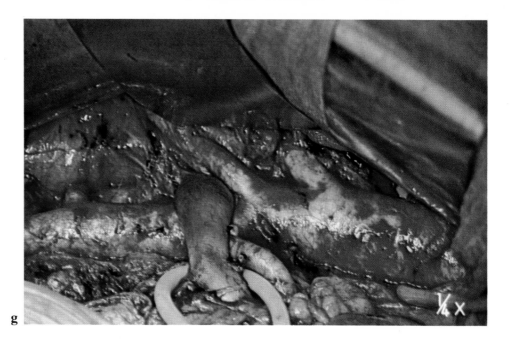

Fig. 5.37 (cont.)   g

146

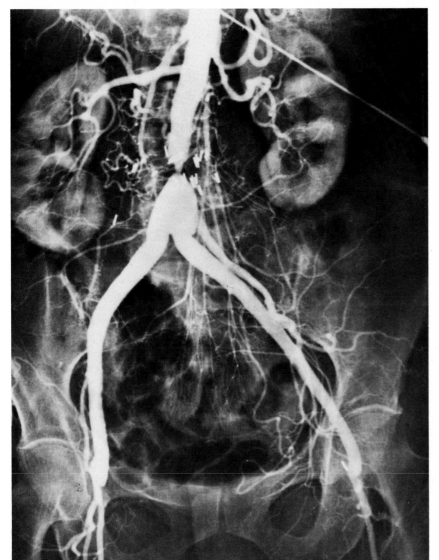

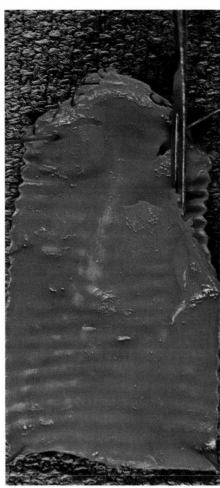

b

a

Fig. 5.38,a, b. Aortogram (a) in a patient who 6 years before had undergone an aorta–bifemoral bypass graft operation for atherosclerotic stenosis which, at that time, was limited to the area of the iliac arteries and the aortic bifurcation. A 22 × 11-mm graft has been anastomosed end-to-side to the aorta at the level of the IMA. During the subsequent years the anticipated progression of atherosclerosis had produced stenosis of the aorta proximal to the graft. Had the original anastomosis to the aorta been made at a more proximal level adjacent to the renal arteries, this complication could have been prevented.

Two additional observations are noteworthy. The tapered narrowing of the aorta between the level of the right renal artery and the zone of extreme stenosis can be anticipated to be due in part to mural thrombus. To avoid embolization, mobilization of this part of the aorta in preparation for installing a new graft requires particular care.

A similar phenomenon has also occurred in the distal portions of the iliac arms of the graft as the result of the use of an oversize graft. The corrugations in the

distal two-thirds of the graft limbs have disappeared, and the lumen in the distal thirds has been reduced by 35% as a result of deposition of mural thrombus. At the second operation, a 12 × 6-mm bifurcation graft was anastomosed end-to-end to the transected infrarenal aorta. The distal limbs of the graft were anastomosed within the abdomen end-to-side to the corresponding segments of the original graft to the corresponding segments of the original graft to preserve flow in the patient's still-patent left common iliac artery.

Two years later disruption of the original left femoral graft anastomosis with a resulting false aneurysm required operative repair. The distal 8 cm of the original graft was replaced with a smaller size graft. **b** The interior of the resected graft. Note the easily detachable pannus of circumferential mural thrombus that lines the interior of the oversize graft. Disruption of this mural thrombus by acute flexion of the thigh is suggested as a possible mechanism in some instances of late graft occlusion following aortofemoral bypass operations.

147

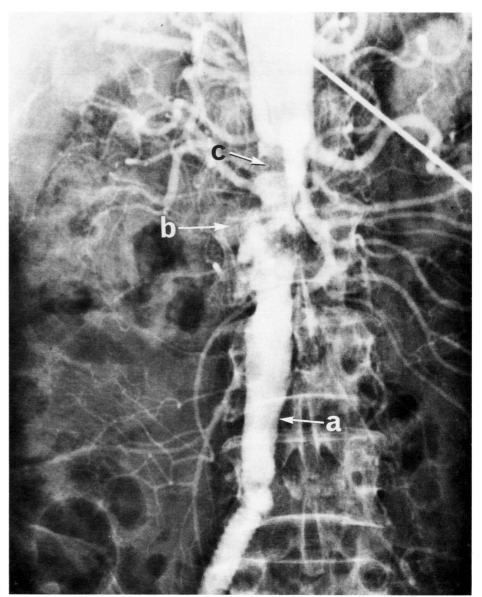

Fig. 5.39a

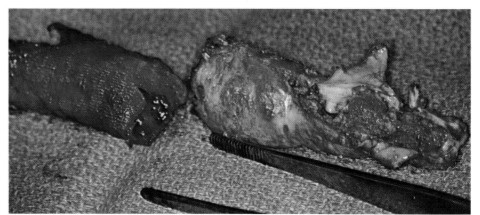

Fig. 5.39b

Fig. 5.39,a, b. Aortogram (**a**) of 61-year-old man with claudication and recent hypertension. Two previous operations had been performed. The first, 18 years before, was a terminal aorta–bilateral common iliac endarterectomy for atherosclerosis limited at that time to the common iliac arteries. Four years later symptoms recurred as a result of obstructing atherosclerotic lesions that had developed at the site of the previous endarterectomy. An aorta–bifemoral bypass grafting operation was performed. The proximal anastomosis was end-to-end to the aorta 5 cm distal to the right renal artery. Minimal intimal thickening was visible in the proximal aortic stump at that time.

The current aortogram shows occlusion of the left iliac limb of the graft. The aortic portion of the graft (*a*) contains a circumferential mural thrombus that narrows its lumen to approximate the size of the patent right iliac limb of the graft. Extensive filling defects are present in the infrarenal aortic stump (*b*) as well as in the suprarenal aorta (*c*).

With a supra SMA aortic clamp in place, an open endarterectomy of the aorta was performed from the SMA to the previous graft anastomosis. Orifice lesions encountered in each of the renal arteries were also removed. The aortic portion of the graft was incised and its contained thrombus removed. A new 14 × 7-mm bifurcation graft was anastomosed to the stump of the aorta, which had been transected 2 cm distal to the right renal artery. The right iliac limb of the graft was anastomosed to the previous graft, and the left iliac limb to the left common femoral artery.

b Endarterectomy specimen and the thrombus removed from the patent aortic portion of the previous graft. The pararenal aorta is almost totally occluded by a massive cauliflower atheroma which extends along one side of the aorta proximal to the renal arteries. Superior to it can be seen the lesion which had been removed from the right renal orifice. The thrombus that was in the graft can be seen to the left.

This case, with its 18-year history of progression of aortoiliac atherosclerosis, illustrates several important aspects of the disease and problems in reconstructive operations.

1. Atherosclerosis which has developed to the degree of arterial occlusion by the early years of the fourth decade has a malignant rate of progression.
2. Atherosclerosis which appears first at the aortic bifurcation area eventually extends to involve the entirety of the infrarenal aorta and rarely, as in this case, the suprarenal aorta as well. The original operation should in every case extend to the renal artery level.
3. Endarterectomized arteries are vulnerable to recurrence of atherosclerosis (but rarely as rapidly as occurred here).
4. The unusual cauliflower type of atherosclerosis or else massive mural thrombus (as in Fig. 7.27) can be anticipated when filling defects of the type shown in this aortogram are observed.
5. Thrombosis of one iliac limb of a bifurcation graft is followed by layering of thrombus in the aortic portion of the graft.

Fig. 5.40,a, b. Aortogram in a patient with left common iliac occlusion and diffuse infrarenal aortic and right common iliac atherosclerosis. The proximal film (**a**) illustrates the pattern of development of atherosclerosis in the aortoiliac segments in which the original lesions appear adjacent to the aortic bifurcation but eventually extend into the full length of the infrarenal aorta. It is this proximal pattern of progression that mandates the selection of the juxtarenal aorta as the site for the cephalad end of the reconstructive operation, whether it be endarterectomy or bypass graft.

The distal film (**b**) reveals a type B pattern of disease. Severe stenosis in the left common femoral artery is obvious. Disease at this site almost invariably occurs in association with lesions in the contralateral common femoral artery and in both external iliac arteries. The barely perceptible irregularities in the right external iliac artery (*a*) and the indentation in the right common femoral artery (*b*) were found at operation to be caused by atherosclerosis. The right renal artery is patent even though not visualized in this study.

Aortography in many patients with type B disease will often show no more than the minimal lesions that appear in this patient's right iliac and common femoral arteries. If a bypass grafting operation is performed one may be tempted to extend the iliac arms of the graft no further than the external iliac arteries if only scattered lesions are palpated at that level. To do so invites recurrence of symptoms as the distal lesions proceed with the inevitable pattern of progression.

At operation on this patient, the profunda femoris arteries were normal. Bilateral common femoral endarterectomy and an aorta–bifemoral grafting procedure were performed.

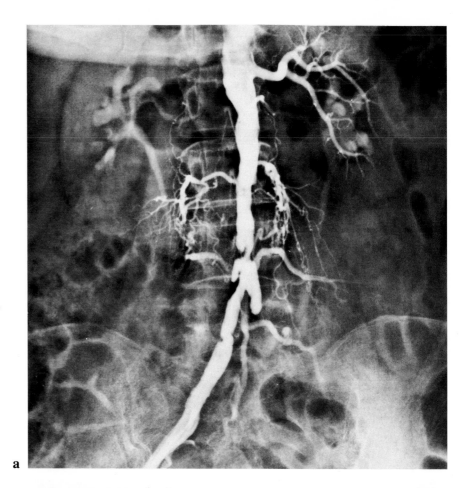

a

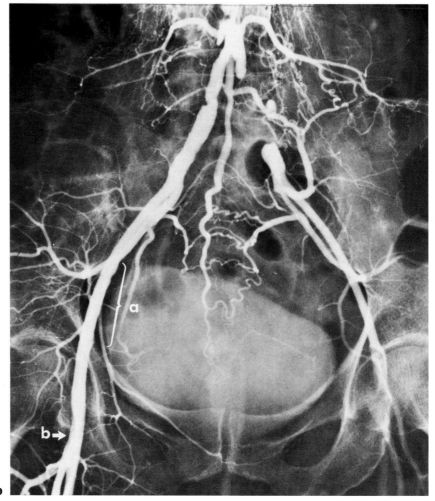

b

150

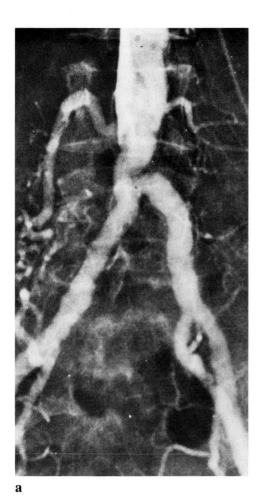

a

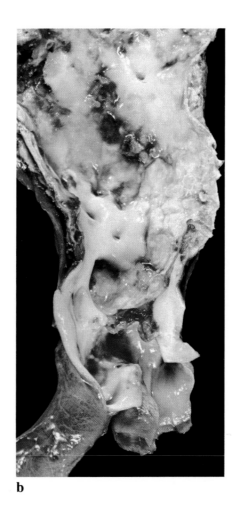

b

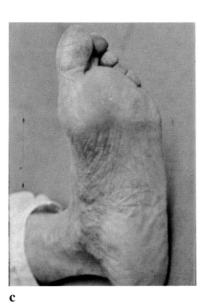

c

Fig. 5.41, a–c.   Blue toe syndrome. Aortogram (**a**), the resected aorta (**b**), and the foot (**c**) in a patient with microemboli to digital arteries. Note the loosely attached atheromatous debris and the scattered mural thrombi in the aortic lumen. Sympathectomy was followed by return of normal color to the cyanotic second toe and resection of the aorta removed the source of further embolization. The friability of the aortic lesion emphasizes the need for gentle mobilization of the aorta and the need for avoiding a reconstructive technique which allows the aorta to remain in the blood flow circuit.

151

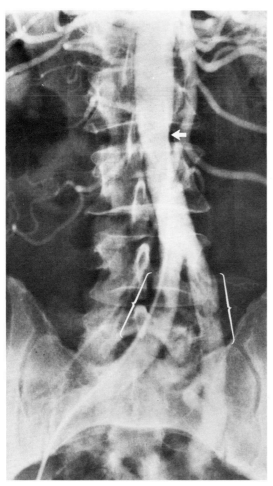

a

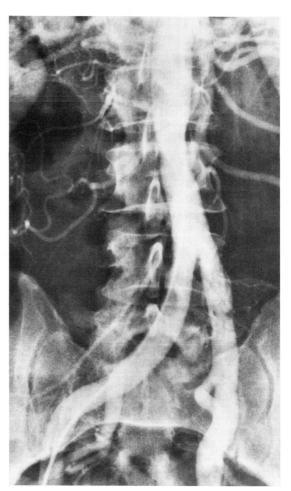

b

Fig. 5.42, a–e. **a, b** Serial films from an aortogram of a 60-year-old man with an acute occlusion of the left popliteal artery culminating eventually in amputation of the leg. Note the barely perceptible indentation of the aorta at the level of the occluded IMA (*arrow*) and the suggestion of filling defects in the common iliac arteries (*brackets*), which were incorrectly diagnosed as overlying bowel shadows. **c, d** Serial films from an aortogram 2 weeks later. Progressive ischemia of the right leg had now developed. Distal films showed stenotic and occlusive lesions at the right popliteal bifurcation not present previously. Note that the narrowing of the aorta has now increased and that the filling defects in the common iliac arteries have become obvious (*arrows*). **e** A lateral projection shows similar filling defects in the terminal aorta. Strings of mural thrombus attached to atheromatous deposits in the wall of the aorta and common iliac arteries were found at operation. The leg was revascularized by popliteal embolectomy.

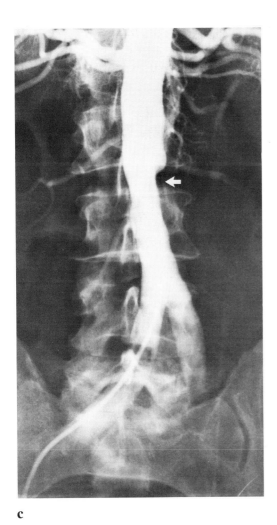

c

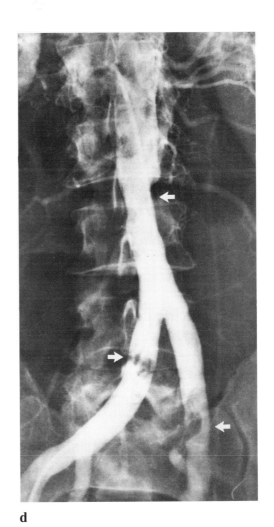

d

Fig. 5.42 (cont.)

e

153

Fig. 5.43. Resected aorta from the patient whose aortograms are shown in Fig. 5.42. The mural thrombus near the center of the specimen was the progressing filling defect seen on the aortogram. Beneath it was found a large atheromatous ulcer. The rope-like thrombus lay free in the aortic lumen attached at both ends to ulcers in the aorta above and in one common iliac artery below. Resection of the aorta and graft replacement were performed to remove the source of further embolization.

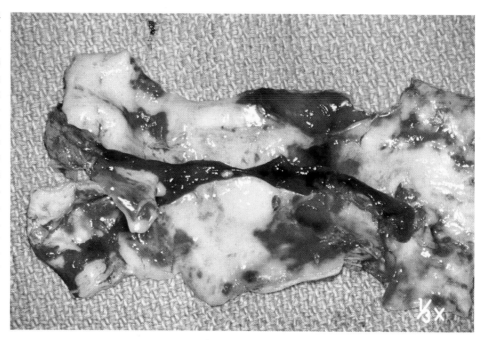

Fig. 5.44,a, b. Aortogram (**a**) in a patient with recurrent emboli to both lower extremities. Note the barely perceptible bulges in the outline of the infrarenal aorta which, by measurement, increased the aortic diameter 2–3 mm beyond that of the suprarenal aorta. **b** Endarterectomy specimen. Degenerative intimal disease and patchy mural thrombus as seen here are often present in portions of the infrarenal aorta where aortography fails to demonstrate the extent of disease. Their presence creates an obvious hazard in the routine employment of partially occluding aortic clamps and the use of end-to-side proximal anastomoses for bypass grafts. Both techniques are condusive to intimal fragmentation and peripheral embolization. In this case, endarterectomy was used because of termination of disease at the common iliac bifurcations. A bypass graft would have given an equally satisfactory result. If a grafting technique is selected in a patient with embolic disease, it is mandatory that it exclude the aortoiliac segment from forward flow by using end-to-end anastomoses at either the proximal or the distal ends of the bypass graft.

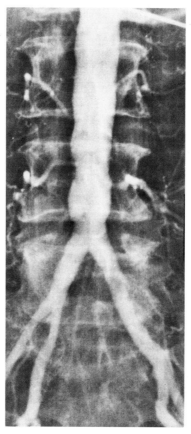

a

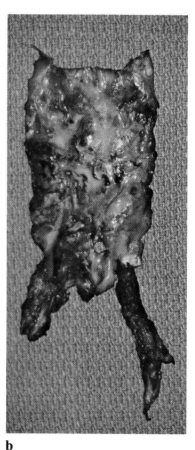

b

154

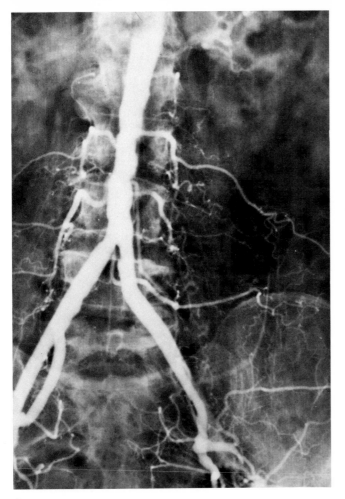

a

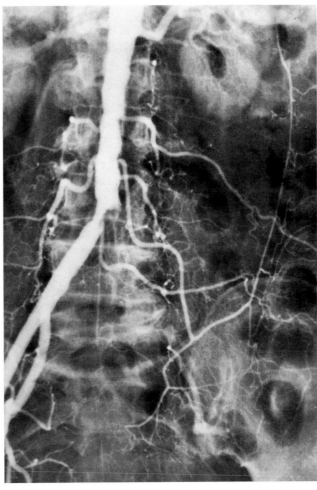

b

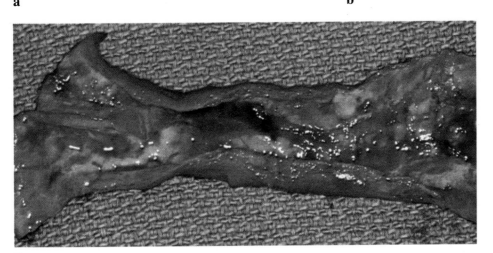

c

Fig. 5.45, a–c. Macroemboli from aortic ASO. **a** Aortogram 24 hours after the onset of acute ischemia in the left leg. The left external iliac artery is occluded and atherosclerotic irregularities are visible in the infrarenal aorta. Operation was refused at this time.

b Aortogram one week later following a sudden increase in left leg ischemia. The left common iliac artery is now occluded and there is a suggestion of thrombus extending upward into the aorta and overflowing into the right common iliac artery. At operation atheroma and loosely attached mural thrombus were found in the aorta. The repeated occlusions in the left iliac system were the result of embolization.

A bifurcation graft was installed with end-to-end anastomoses to the justarenal aorta and to the right common iliac artery and an end-to-side anastomosis to the left common femoral artery. Iliac thrombectomy was not attempted because of uncertainty concerning possible atheroma in the left external iliac artery. A bypass graft with an end-to-side anastomosis to the aorta would have been hazardous to install and would have left the patient vulnerable to embolization to the right leg.

c Resected aorta. Note the thrombus loosely attached to atheromatous plaques.

155

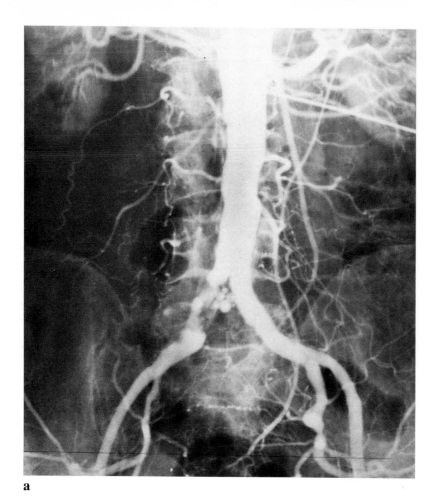

a

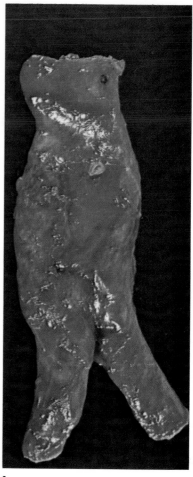

b

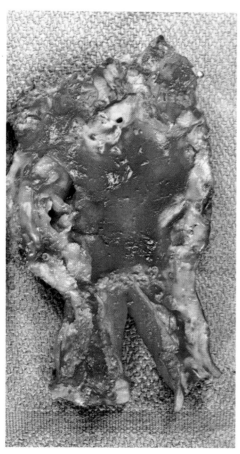

c

Fig. 5.46,a–c. Aortogram (**a**) of a patient with atherosclerotic stenosis of the right common iliac artery. The contour of the iliac lumen and the slight irregular widening of the infrarenal aorta indicates the type of patulous arterial degeneration often associated with granular decomposition of the intima. Mobilization should be performed with particular care to prevent distal embolization. Bypass grafting with an infrarenal end-to-end anastomosis is preferable to endarterectomy or an end-to-side bypass graft.

Photographs of the resected infrarenal aorta. The enlarged and patulous aorta (**b**) observed at laparotomy suggested extensive intimal disease in the aorta. The opened specimen (**c**) shows degeneration and thickening of the aortic wall and extensive mural thrombus, both of which combined to produce the aortographic contour of an almost normal-appearing aorta.

156

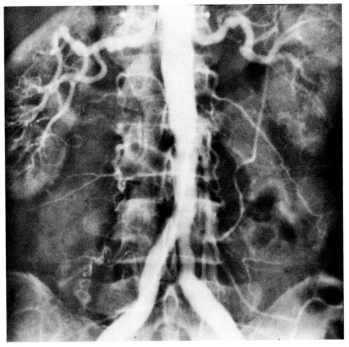

a

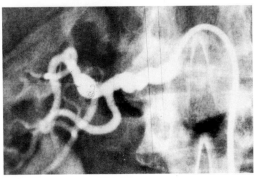

b

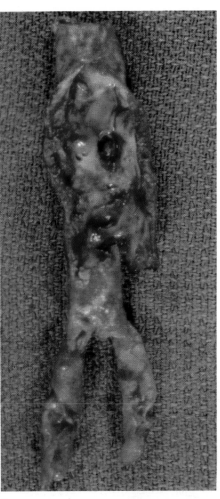

c

Fig. 5.47. **a** Aortogram in a 52-year-old woman with what appears to be minimal and nonobstructing atherosclerotic irregularities in the infrarenal aorta and fibromuscular dysplasia of the right renal artery. The latter lesion is best shown by the selective renal arteriogram (**b**).

The primary objective of operation was to relieve hypertension by means of a graft from the aorta to the distal right renal artery. It was suspected that there would be generalized atherosclerosis in the aorta, which would make it unsuitable for a proximal anastomosis. This problem was overcome by performing a preliminary aortoiliac endarterectomy.

Endarterectomy specimen (**c**) illustrates the gross degenerative intimal disease, and even mural thrombus, that can be present and not be revealed in an aortogram. The frequent existence of lesions such as these in aortic atherosclerosis illustrates the care that must be exercised to prevent embolization from the aortic wall during mobilization of an atherosclerotic aorta. The same hazard is also present in other patients with obstructive atherosclerosis of the aortic bifurcation and an apparently nondiseased infrarenal aortic segment for whom a bypass grafting operation with a proximal end-to-side anastomosis is planned. The installation of a graft onto the side of an atherosclerotic aorta creates the added hazard of intimal fragmentation at the site of clamp application and subsequent embolization when the clamps are removed.

In the endarterectomy specimen, note the granular degeneration in the aortic wall, the intimal ulceration, and, near the bifurcation, the mural thrombus in the lumen. The aortic endarterectomy had been performed for the dual purpose of preventing later aortic occlusion and providing an aortic wall to which a bypass graft to one or both renal arteries can safely be anastomosed. The appearance of the specimen emphasizes the care that must be taken in mobilizing or clamping the abdominal aorta when any degree of irregularity is visible by aortography.

157

Aortic
Aneurysms

6

Unruptured Infrarenal Aortic Aneurysms

Atherosclerotic aneurysmal disease of the abdominal aorta in its most common form involves the segment of the aorta distal to the renal arteries and, to a variable degree, the common iliac arteries as well. Aortic dilatation usually begins 3–5 cm beyond the renal artery orifices, with the segment between the renal arteries and the beginning of the aneurysm usually having a normal external diameter. The intima in this segment may undergo variable degrees of atherosclerotic degeneration, but the media and adventitia retain adequate strength to hold a suture line for graft anastomosis. The long-term integrity of the aortic wall does not extend beyond the first 3–5 cm of the infrarenal aorta. Occasionally the aneurysm will involve only a more distal segment of the infrarenal aorta. It is important to recognize that, in this case, aortic dilatation at a higher level will develop in time and that aortic transection in preparation for graft replacement should be done at the customary level immediately distal to the renal arteries.

Anatomy

Since an increase in aortic diameter is also accompanied by increase in length, the aortic bifurcation is thus projected distally beyond the normal L_4 level. Similar elongation of the common iliac arteries results in tortuosity and frequent dislocation of their bifurcations into the depths of the pelvis. Proximally the elongation of the infrarenal aorta may dislocate its proximal end to one side or the other, and anteriorly as well. As the expanding aneurysm carries the afferent portion of the aorta anterior to its usual position, the perirenal segment of the undilated aorta becomes a continuation of the palpable convexity of the anterior surface of the aneurysmal infrarenal aorta. To the uninitiated, palpation of the retroperitoneal mass before its components have been dissected often leads to an erroneous diagnosis of aneurysmal involvement of the suprarenal aorta. The frequent anterior dislocation of the infrarenal nonaneurysmal segment of the aorta often provides a space between the aorta and the vertebral bodies through which finger dissection encounters minimal or no resistance.

159

The inferior mesenteric artery (IMA), which has its origin on the left anterolateral surface of the aorta, often becomes flattened, elongated, and partially imbedded in the aortic wall as the aneurysm enlarges. Its left colic branch is a major source of collateral to the left transverse and proximal descending colon from the superior mesenteric artery after the IMA has been ligated at its origin; it may arise from the imbedded portion of the IMA and must be carefully preserved during unroofing of the aneurysm.

With large aneurysms, the fourth portion of the duodenum becomes flattened against the right side of the aneurysm. The medial edge of the duodenum should be carefully identified before the retroperitoneal incision is made. The interior of the aorta in the area of the aneurysm is usually lined by a 1–4 cm layer of laminated thrombus. The functioning lumen of the aorta, surrounded by a thick, jellylike layer of thrombus, may have a normal diameter. A similar phenomenon is frequently encountered in dilated portions of the common iliac arteries. During mobilization of these arterial segments, particular care should be taken to avoid disruption and fragmentation of the anticipated thrombus within (**Fig. 6.1a and b**).

Atherosclerotic thickening of the wall of the common iliac artery is present in varying degrees. This becomes maximum at the iliac bifurcation, where calcification is often encountered. The external iliac arteries uniformly undergo a mild degree of cylindrical dilatation. Mural thrombus and atherosclerotic thickening of the arterial wall, however, are rarely encountered, a fact of some significance in selecting the site for distal attachment of a graft.

Abdominal Incision

Laparotomy is most expeditiously accomplished through a full-length midline incision from the xyphoid process to the symphysis pubis (**Fig. 6.2**). A shorter incision requires excessive muscle retraction to accomplish ade-

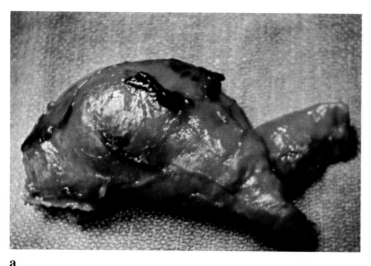
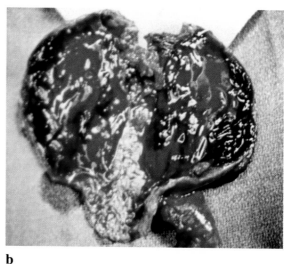

a   b

Fig. 6.1. **a** A resected 7-cm aortic aneurysm in a patient with a recent embolus to one popliteal artery. **b** The thick mural thrombus within the aneurysm, thought to be the source of the embolus, varies from the usual thrombus in that it appears to be fresh and particularly friable. The usual thrombus is darker in color with a stable gelatinous consistency and a smooth luminal surface that rarely embolizes except as the result of direct trauma.

160

quate exposure of the infrarenal aorta superiorly and the bifurcation of the common iliac arteries inferiorly. A transverse abdominal incision to provide access to the aorta, either transperitoneally or retroperitoneally, is often adequate and lessens the postoperative incisional pain. We have tended not to use this incision, however, because it may limit exposure substantially if an unanticipated problem is encountered.

The small intestines are encased in a plastic bag and brought out onto the abdominal wall to the right of the incision. The posterior peritoneal incision is made longitudinally on the dome of the aneurysm to the right of the vascular arcade supplying the left colon (**Fig. 6.3**). It is deepened through the periaortic soft tissue to the adventitia, at which level a relatively avascular dissection plane can be developed. The incision is extended superiorly to the left renal vein in a line midway between the medial edge of the duodenum and the inferior mesenteric vein. To improve exposure, the inferior mesenteric vein may be safely transected as it crosses the neck of the aneurysm. Inferiorly the retroperitoneal incision swings to the right over the anterior surface of the right common iliac artery to avoid the medially situated branches of the IMA extending into the pelvis.

The anterior two-thirds of the aneurysm is then unroofed, separating it from the duodenum on the right to the depth of the inferior vena cava

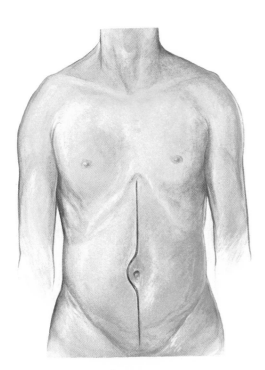

Fig. 6.2. Preferred laparotomy incision for aortic aneurysmectomy.

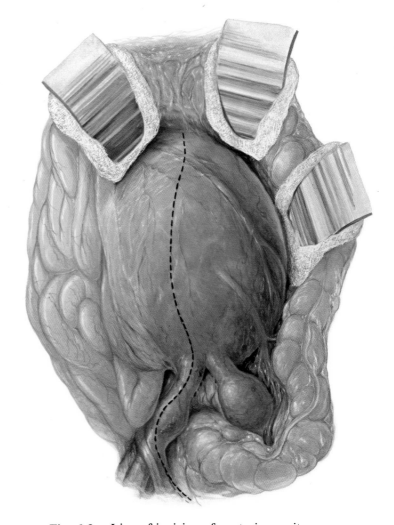

Fig. 6.3. Line of incision of posterior peritoneum.

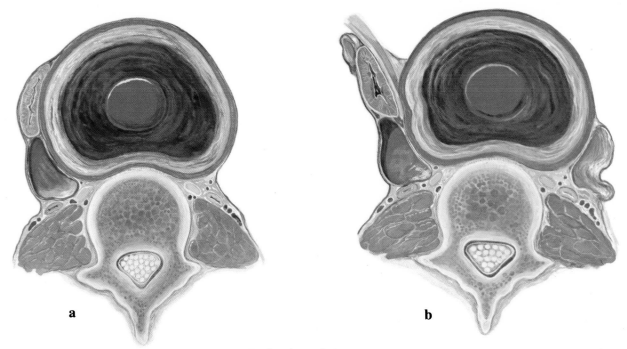

Fig. 6.4,a, b. Reflection of duodenum. **a** customary relation of duodenum to wall of aneurysm; **b** mobilization of duodenum to level of vena cava.

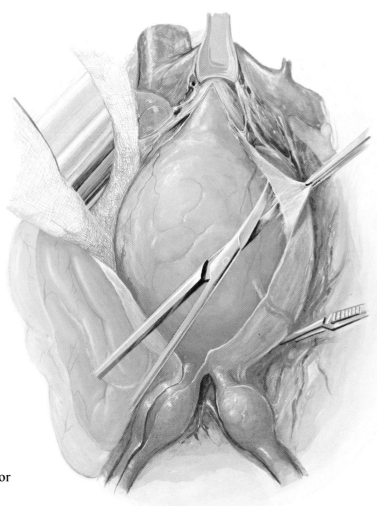

Fig. 6.5. Denuding anterior surface of aneurysm.

162

(**Fig. 6.4a and b**). The plane of dissection is illustrated in **Fig. 6.5**. The left renal vein has been retracted superiorly. The layer of fibrous disease surrounding the proximal aorta above the upper end of the aneurysm has been incised by an extension of the original midline incision. Preservation of this layer as the proximal aorta is mobilized is particularly important since this is the tissue that will be used to cover the aorta–graft anastomosis.

Iliac Mobilization

Mobilization of the distal right common iliac artery is started from its midpoint on the right side where the right common iliac vein is in clear view (**Fig. 6.6a and b**). Both of the common iliac veins course to the right of the respective iliac arteries, and mobilization of the left common iliac artery should begin from its right surface also. Initiation of the dissection of the iliac artery origins adjacent to the aortic bifurcation is particularly hazard-

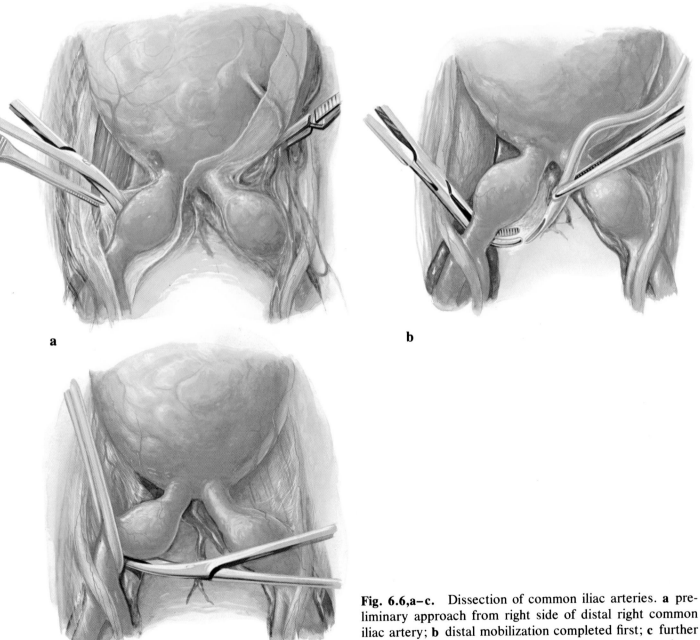

a

b

c

Fig. 6.6,a–c. Dissection of common iliac arteries. **a** preliminary approach from right side of distal right common iliac artery; **b** distal mobilization completed first; **c** further mobilization limited to segment needed for anastomosis.

163

ous and should not be attempted at this stage. Bleeding from laceration of the caval bifurcation behind the iliac arteries is particularly difficult to control without excessive blood loss. Once slings have been passed behind the iliac arteries, the posterior mobilization can be performed with greater safety (**Fig. 6.6c**).

Exposure of the anterior surface of the left common iliac artery is developed by finger dissection in a plane on the surface of the artery (**Fig. 6.7a**). This relatively avascular dissection plane lies posterior to both the mesenteric vasculature and the left ureter. Note that the right-sided position of the original retroperitoneal incision permits preservation of the midline portion of the vascular arcade in the sigmoid mesentery. Special considerations in exposure of the left common iliac artery may be advisable in the sexually active male (see p. 111).

Since clamp control of both external iliac hypogastric arteries will often be required, all four should be skeletonized and encircled with rubber tubing. Exposure of the left common iliac bifurcation and the external iliac and hypogastric arteries is usually facilitated by an approach through the left iliac fossa after medial reflection of the sigmoid colon (**Fig. 6.7b**).

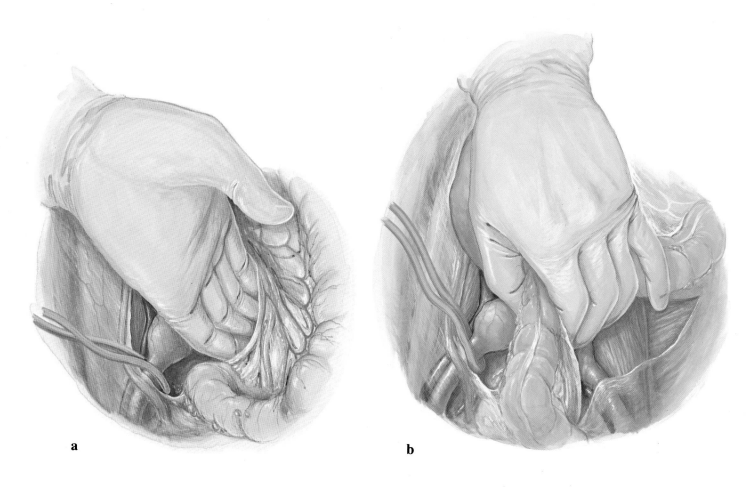

a   b

Fig. 6.7, a, b. Exposure of left iliac bifurcation. **a** manual dissection from midline along surface of artery; **b** distal dissection by reflection of sigmoid colon.

Preparation of Proximal Aorta

The final maneuvers are directed toward mobilization of the proximal aorta to the level of the renal arteries. The anterior two-thirds of the surface of the aorta can be skeletonized under direct vision. Some degree of retraction of the lateral wall of the aneurysm at its proximal end may be necessary. Retraction should be spread over a broad area with four fingers on a folded laparotomy tape (**Fig. 6.8a**). The use of a sponge on a clamp or a single finger for this purpose risks perforation of the aneurysm. Specially designed deep, narrow retractors with a curved flange to prevent tearing of the vessels behind it are particularly valuable during this portion of the dissection (**Fig. 6.8b**).

Several small arterial branches from the side of the aorta, including the gonadal arteries, will be encountered as the dissection is deepened and should be individually divided and tied. If a larger arterial branch of the aorta is encountered, its termination should be identified before ligation since it may be a branch of the lower pole of the kidney. A lower pole artery arising proximal to the beginning of the aneurysm should be preserved. If it originates at the beginning of or from the wall of the aneurysm and if it is small in comparison to the main renal artery, it may be safely ligated. Infarction of a small segment of the lower pole of the kidney will result, but this event is more benign than is placing the graft anastomosis in the proximal portion of the aneurysmal wall in an effort to preserve the polar artery. If the accessory renal artery is equal in size to an ipsilateral renal artery proximal to it, it should be preserved for later anastomosis to the side of the graft. Rarely a single renal artery may have a low origin and require reimplantation.

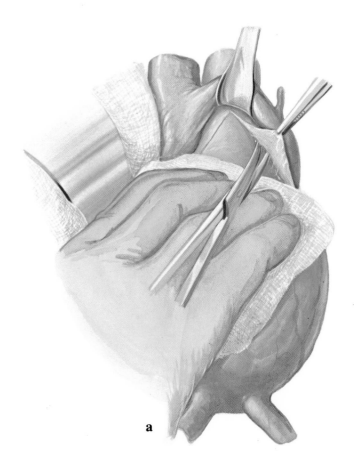

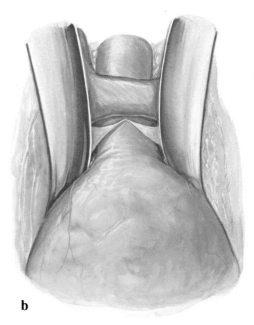

Fig. 6.8,a, b. Dissection of proximal aorta. **a** retraction of proximal end of aneurysm; **b** renal vein retractors for exposure of infrarenal aorta.

The final potential difficulty at this stage of the mobilization is the seldom encountered retroaortic left renal vein. Except for the patient with congenital absence of the left kidney, one can be certain of its presence if the aortic dissection fails to expose the vein in its usual anterior position. Rarely the renal vein will bifurcate with one branch passing behind the aorta.

The posterior third of the proximal aorta is mobilized by blunt finger dissection. **Fig. 6.9a** depicts the space behind the aorta that has been created by the aneurysm. The lumbar arteries can be palpated as taut strands. Gentle manipulation of the dissecting finger will develop a plane between successive pairs of lumbar arteries adjacent to the origin of the renal arteries (**Fig. 6.9b**). If substantial resistance is encountered, this maneuver should be abandoned in favor of proceeding with an alternate technique (Fig. 6.24a, b; see p. 179).

Technique

Fig. 6.10a illustrates the beginning stage of operation in the pathologic situation most frequently encountered (variations in this pattern often occur and will be described later). There is a short segment of nonaneurysmal aorta distal to the renal arteries. Aneurysmal disease in the common iliac arteries is present, but spares the portion proximal to their bifurcation. The distal common iliac arteries are free of calcific or occlusive atherosclerosis.

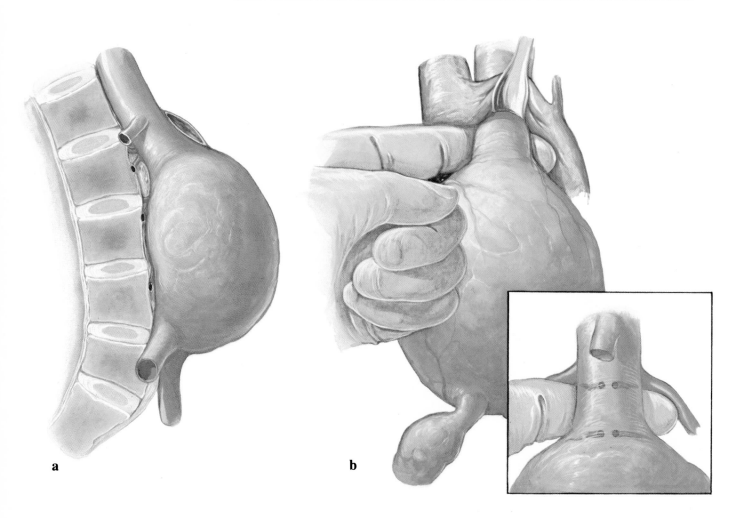

a   b

Fig. 6.9,a, b. Mobilization of proximal aorta. **a** anterior dislocation of perirenal aorta by growth of aneurysm; **b** finger dissection between lumbar arteries.

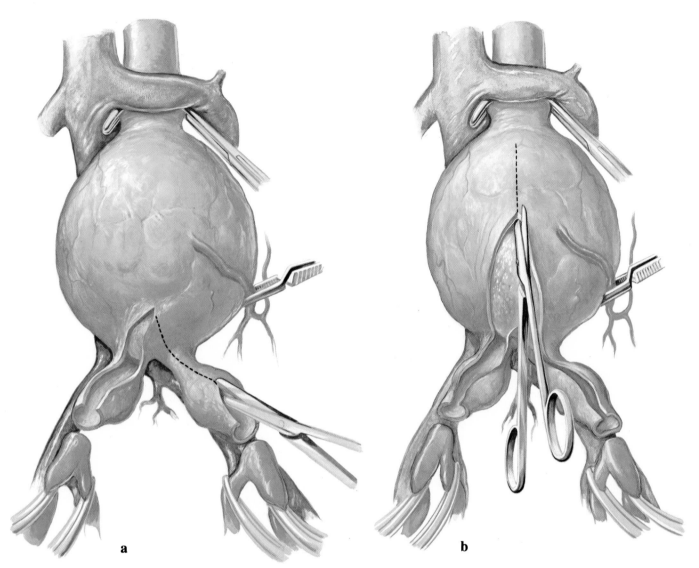

Fig. 6.10,a, b. Aortotomy. **a** distal; **b** proximal extent of original incision.

The proximal aortic clamp is applied as closely as possible to the origins of the renal arteries without impinging upon their orifices. A bulldog clamp has been applied to the inferior mesenteric artery. The hypogastric and external iliac arteries have been individually clamped. The clamps used on these arteries have been designed with a long, slightly curved blade to permit their application from outside the abdominal cavity and an angulated shank to allow the handles to lie flat on the abdominal wall. Clamps are not applied to the common iliac arteries unless they are palpably free of disease in order to avoid intima–media disruption at a site that may become the one most suitable for graft anastomosis.

Incision of Aneurysm　The aneurysm is opened through a longitudinal incision extending proximally on the right side of the inferior mesenteric artery orifice (**Fig. 6.10b**). This exposes the exterior surface of the laminated clot that almost invariably surrounds the aortic lumen. A small volume of murky, purulent-appearing (but sterile) liquid may escape at this time. At this stage the proximal aortotomy is extended to a level just caudad to the anticipated level for transection of the aorta.

A left lateral extension of the aortotomy may be made to surround the orifice of the inferior mesenteric artery to permit this artery and a narrow cuff of adjacent aortic wall to be set aside for later evaluation of collateral backbleeding. A simpler technique for this purpose, however, is to observe backbleeding from the orifice of the undivided IMA from within the aneurysm after completion of the graft anastomoses. If, at this time, backbleeding is inadequate and if there is evidence of left colon ischemia, the IMA may be anastomosed to the graft. (**Fig. 6.11a and b**). It is important to note, however, that when safeguards are taken to preserve the vasculature in the left colon, adequate collateral blood supply is almost invariably present. Reimplantation of the IMA into the graft is rarely necessary. If encountered, a large renal polar branch arising from the wall of the aneurysm should be removed along with a cuff of aortic wall. It is reimplanted onto the graft as soon as the proximal aortic anastomosis has been accomplished (**Fig. 6.12a–c**).

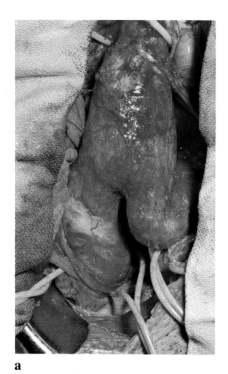

a

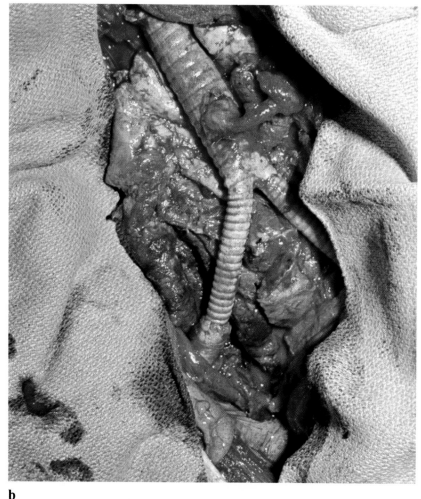

b

Fig. 6.11,a, b. Implantation of IMA. **a** Exposed aneurysm at laparotomy. **b** Aortic bifurcation graft in place to which has been anastomosed the IMA. Note the residual wall of the aneurysm that will be wrapped around the prosthesis.

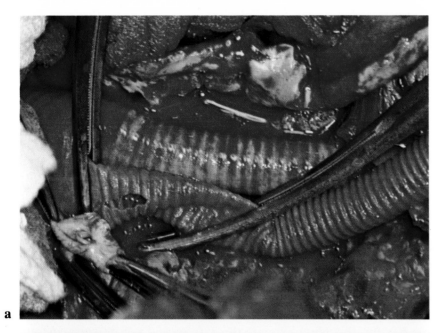

a

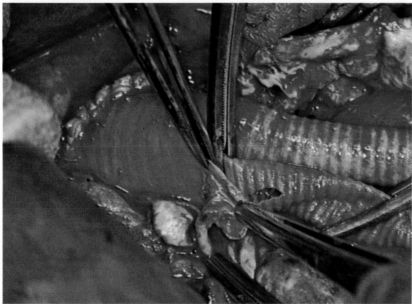

b

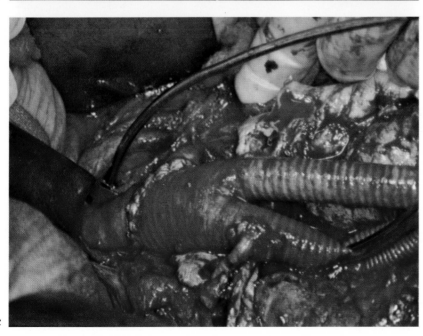

c

Fig. 6.12,a–c. Anastomosis of the right renal artery to the right iliac arm of a prosthetic graft using the Carrel patch technique. Operation was performed for the management of a large atherosclerotic aneurysm extending upward to the renal artery level. The upper level of the aneurysm was at the origin of the left renal artery. The right renal artery originated from the aneurysm at a more distal level. The proximal aortic clamp was placed proximal to the left renal artery and the aorta was transected at a level providing a 2-cm cuff for the proximal anastomosis. **a** An opening has been made in the side of the right iliac limb of the graft (patient's head to the left). Note the detached right renal artery with a flange of aortic wall. **b** Flange positioned for anastomosis. The left renal vein and the proximal anastomosis can be seen to the left. **c** Completed renal anastomosis.

169

The contained thrombus is removed manually and is delivered as a globular, jellylike bolus (**Fig. 6.13a**). Backbleeding from the lumbar arteries may be profuse and is controlled before proceeding further. The orifices of these arteries are usually surrounded by a thick layer of calcified aortic intima, which must be removed by a local endarterectomy to permit suture closure. Small, figure-of-eight transfixion sutures will firmly seal each bleeding orifice (**Fig. 6.13b**).

Anticoagulation Systemic heparinization is deferred until completion of the aortic graft anastomosis in order to assure prompt sealing of the proximal suture line, assuming that no unusual problems are anticipated and that the surgeon has the experience needed for rapid performance of this anastomosis. During the 10–15 min of aortic occlusion required for completion of this portion of the operation, the only arterial segments vulnerable to intraluminal thrombosis are the external iliac arteries, which contain a static column of blood to the level of their respective inferior epigastric and circumflex iliac branches. The return of blood into the distal arterial tree beyond this level extends the safe period before spontaneous thrombosis occurs in the distal vessels. After the demonstration of adequate backbleeding following release of the external iliac clamps, the blood in the external iliac segment is displaced by perfusion with dilute heparin solution (**Fig. 6.14**).

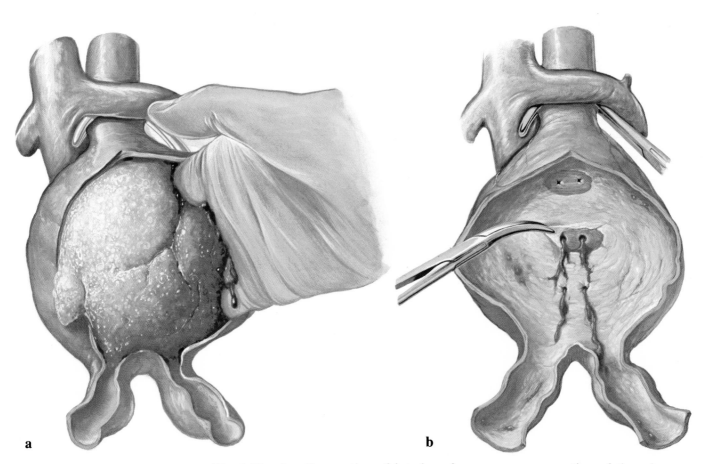

a   b

Fig. 6.13,a, b. Preparation of interior of aneurysm. **a** vacuation of thrombus; **b** closure of lumbar arteries.

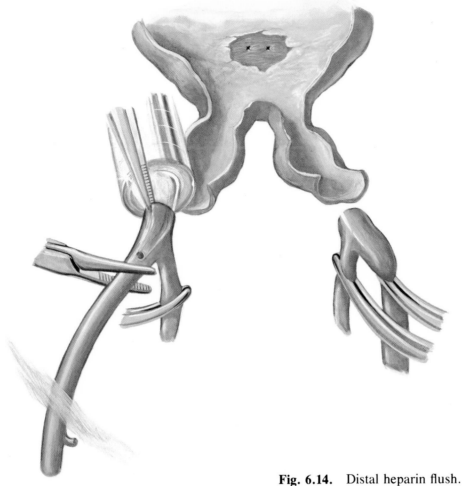

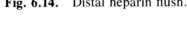

Fig. 6.14. Distal heparin flush.

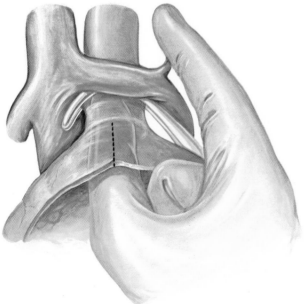

Fig. 6.15. Palpation of the aortic ring, if present, at origin of aneurysm to determine level of transection.

Proximal Anastomosis   Attention is now directed to the proximal end. Insertion of a thumb into the proximal aorta will usually allow one to palpate the level of the beginning of the aneurysm (**Fig. 6.15**). The aortotomy is then extended to this level and the aorta transected. The characteristic ringlike impediment to the further insertion of the thumb will not be encountered when aneurysmal degeneration extends proximally in the aorta to the level of the renal arteries. This situation can usually be anticipated during mobilization of the infrarenal aorta. If a normal-sized segment of the aorta distal to the renal arteries is not observed, it is preferable to clamp the aorta proximal to the renal arteries and to transect the infrarenal aorta as close to the renal arteries as possible, preserving only enough of a cuff to contain the anastomotic sutures. The intima of the aorta at the level of the renal arteries in aneurysms that begin at this level is frequently degenerated, and it is often prudent to place the proximal aortic clamp at a supraceliac level. Aneurysms beginning at this level are usually large, and access to the supraceliac aorta may be difficult to obtain. The use of a sternum-elevating retractor substantially improves the exposure (**Fig. 6.16a and b**).

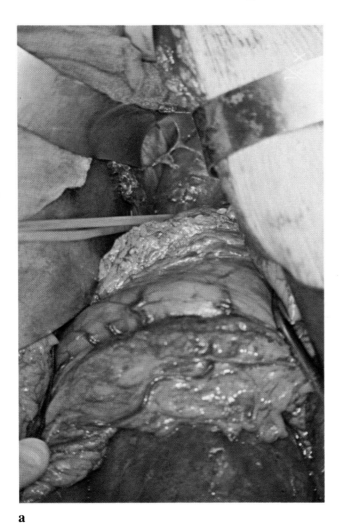 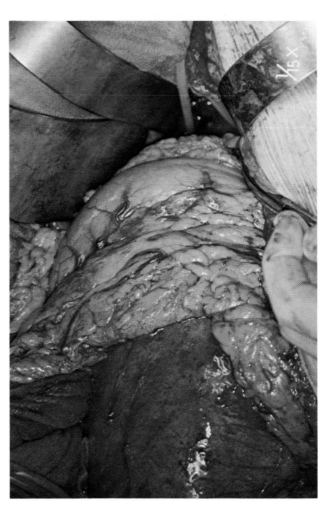

a   b

Fig. 6.16,a, b. Clamp occlusion of the supraceliac aorta from the abdominal approach is frequently desirable in various reconstructive operations involving the abdominal aorta and its major branches in the upper abdomen. Forceful elevation of the lower sternum aids in obtaining the necessary exposure. These photographs were taken during the course of an operation on a patient with an abdominal aneurysm (visible at bottom of photographs). The unusually cephalad position of the aneurysm required transection of the aorta at a level that would allow a graft anastomosis within a few mm of the renal artery orifices. Suprarenal clamping of the aorta is, therefore, necessary. Exposure and mobilization of the supraceliac aorta is easier and safer to accomplish than periaortic dissection in the restricted zone subjacent to the SMA.

a The supraceliac aorta is encircled with latex tubing preparatory to crossclamping. The sternum has been elevated with a Goligher sternal retractor (partially seen at top). The posterior fibers of the diaphragm have been split (upper left). The tubing encircles the aorta proximal to the celiac artery. **b** Restricted exposure in the absence of sternal elevation.

Whether the aneurysm begins adjacent to or more distal to the renal arteries, the intima in the infrarenal aortic segment will have undergone variable degrees of atherosclerotic degeneration and fragmentation but without substantial thickening. Only rarely does it become necessary to endarterectomize this segment to remove grossly thickened intima. The outer aortic wall is usually strong and not calcified. Loose material in the lumen is removed by vigorous flushing (**Fig. 6.17**). Close, deeply placed sutures for the graft anastomosis adequately bind less loosely attached intimal fragments that remain.

In our experience the preferred graft replacement technique is one that utilizes a bifurcation graft. The use of a tube graft, favored by some surgeons because of the propinquity of the two iliac orifices, makes it necessary to use a diseased aortic wall for creation of the distal anastomosis. The possibility of immediate or late failure from intimal disruption or thrombosis when a tube graft is anastomosed to the distal aorta is greater than if the iliac arms of a bifurcation graft were available for anastomosis to less diseased distal arterial segments.

The aortic portion of the graft is transected 3–4 cm from its bifurcation and anastomosed to the aortic stump. The resulting high bifurcation permits greater flexibility in aligning the course of the iliac arms of the graft to adopt to the fixed position of the recipient iliac arteries distally.

The commercially available grafts provide a 2:1 ratio between the diameters of the aortic and iliac segments. In aneurysmal disease this precise ratio between the diameters of the infrarenal aorta and the common iliac arteries is rarely encountered. Selection of the most appropriate graft should favor the graft that has an aortic segment that most closely approximates the size of the proximal aorta (usually 14–16 mm). Adjustments to overcome size disparities are safer and easier to accomplish in the iliac anastomoses. In most cases, a 16 × 8 or a 14 × 7 graft will provide an aortic end of appropriate diameter.

For the aortic anastomosis we prefer the 4–0 multifilament coated Ti-Cron double-ended suture, with T-16 needles. For the right-handed surgeon, a single-layer continuous closure is begun at the four o'clock posi-

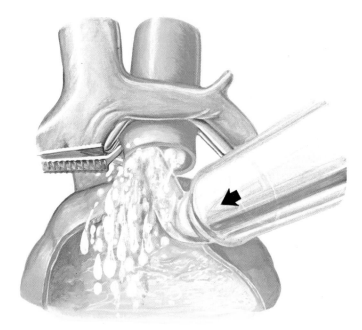

Fig. 6.17. Irrigation debridement of aortic stump.

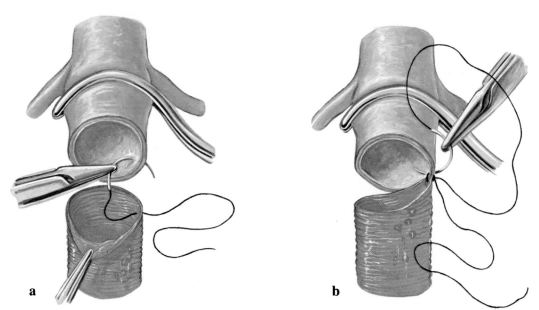

a   b

Fig. 6.18,a, b. Beginning of graft anastomosis. **a** first suture at 4 o'clock position; **b** suture returned into aortic lumen.

tion on the aortic stump with the knot on the outside (**Fig. 6.18a**). The needle is reinserted into the aorta from the outside to prepare for suturing the posterior layer from an inside approach (**Fig. 6.18b**). Deeply placed "bites" on the aortic side are advisable in order to obtain a tight and strong seal. The interior approach is terminated at the nine o'clock position, and the anterior layer is completed from the conventional outside approach using the other end of the suture (**Fig. 6.19a and b**).

The graft is given a quick flush by momentary release of the aortic clamp to wash away disrupted intimal fragments contained within the jaws of the clamp. The entire graft is then held upward to expose the posterior suture line, and after finger compression of the iliac arms the aortic clamp is again released. Even with careful preclotting, diffuse ooze through the interstices of the customarily used knitted graft will be observed. The purpose of this maneuver is to identify inadvertent gaps in the suture line that can be effectively closed after reapplication of the clamp with one or more supplemental sutures (**Fig. 6.20a**).

Distal Anastomosis   With the aortic clamp closed (not shown in drawing), liquid blood within the graft is removed by milking the iliac arms, following which dilute heparin is instilled into the graft without pressure (**Fig. 6.20b**). The slight loss of the preclotting effect is more than balanced by the assurance that intragraft thrombus will not develop while the distal anastomoses are being established. It is advisable not to replace the original aorta clamp with individual clamps on the iliac arms of the graft at this time. The blood in the resulting infrarenal cul-de-sac is particularly susceptible to thrombosis during the time the iliac anastomoses are being completed.

Aortic occlusion time for this portion of the operation rarely exceeds 10–15 min, a generally safe time interval before distal intra-arterial thrombosis begins to develop. Systemic heparinization is now induced for protection during the longer period for completing the iliac anastomoses. A single dose of 3500 units will produce the necessary effect for the additional 15–20 min before all clamps have been released. If a longer time interval should occur, supplemental heparin is given (1500 units for each additional 30 min of arterial occlusion).

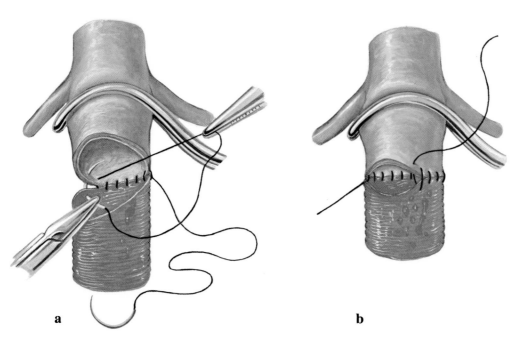

a   b

Fig. 6.19,a, b. Completion of anastomosis. **a** posterior sutures; **b** anterior sutures.

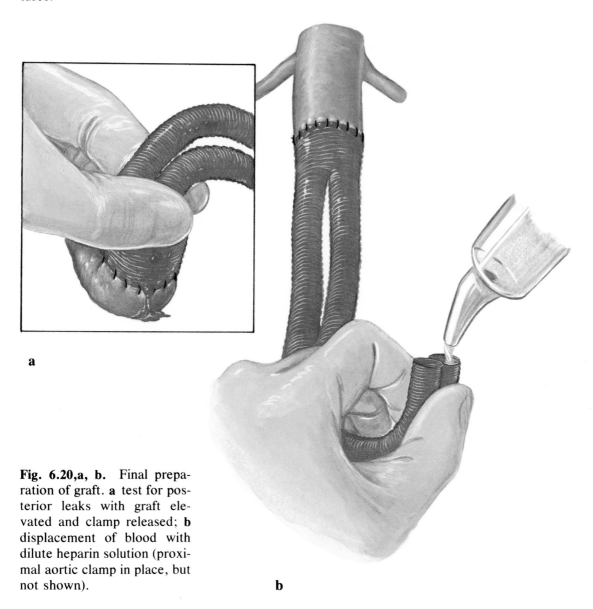

a

Fig. 6.20,a, b. Final preparation of graft. **a** test for posterior leaks with graft elevated and clamp released; **b** displacement of blood with dilute heparin solution (proximal aortic clamp in place, but not shown).

b

175

The iliac anastomoses are made with 5–0 Ti-Cron using a technique on the posterior suture line similar to that used for the aortic anastomosis. In the common pathologic situation described above, most of the circumference of the iliac intima is pliable and adaptable for using "make-up" suture placement to overcome a disparity in graft size. Before completion of the first anastomosis, selective release of the proximal aortic and distal iliac clamps assures inflow and outflow patency.

Clamp Release   A final flush through the unsutured opposite iliac arm of the graft by momentary release of the aortic clamp removes clotted blood that may have accumulated on the aortic cul-de-sac (**Fig. 6.21a**). As in com-

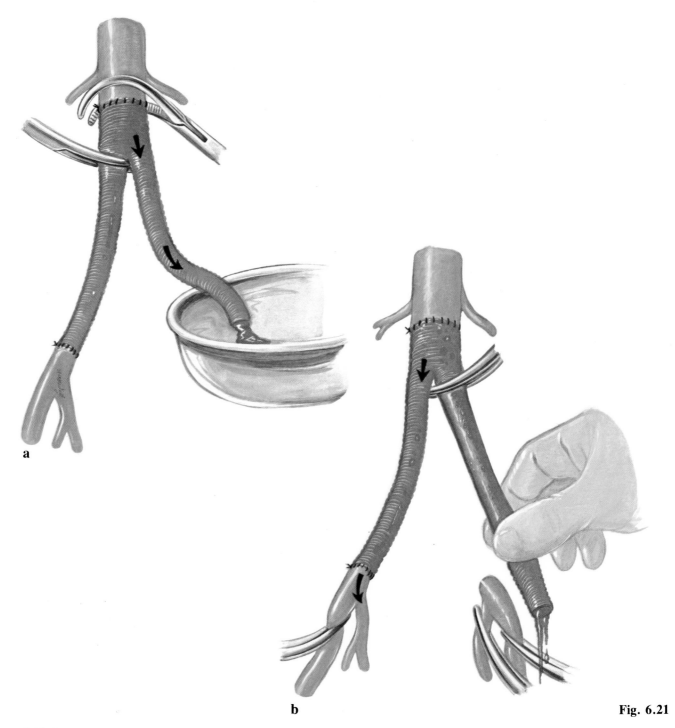

a

b

Fig. 6.21

176

parable situation elsewhere, forward flow into the anastomosed side is opened first to an arterial branch supplying an area least likely to cause difficulty if embolization were to occur—in this case, the outflow tract of the hypogastric artery (**Fig. 6.21b**). A momentary fall in blood pressure may occur; it should return to normal in 1–2 min. At this time, the external iliac clamp is released (**Fig. 6.21c**).

Following completion of the opposite iliac anastomosis, similar staged release of the distal clamps is performed (**Fig. 6.21d**). If blood and third-space losses have been adequately compensated, the successive release of each of the four distal occluding clamps will rarely cause more than a transient 10–20 mm Hg fall in systemic blood pressure.

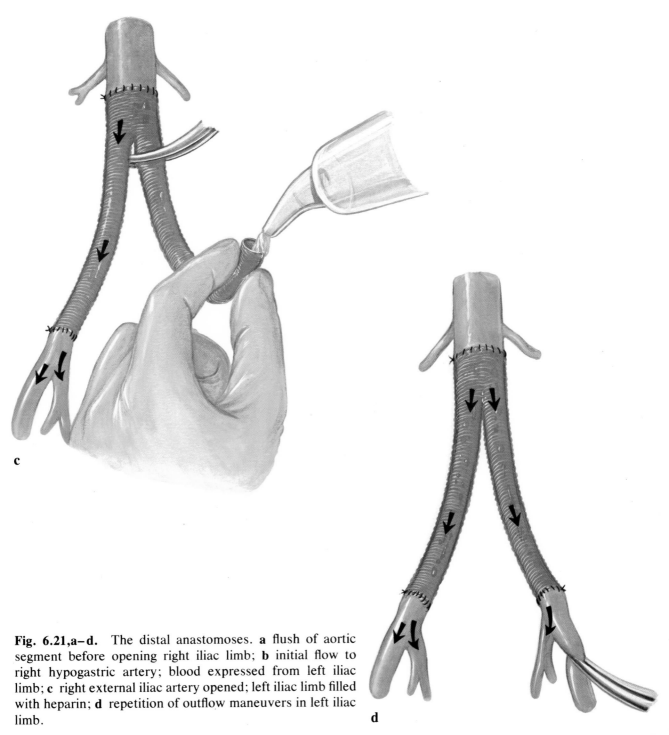

Fig. 6.21,a–d. The distal anastomoses. **a** flush of aortic segment before opening right iliac limb; **b** initial flow to right hypogastric artery; blood expressed from left iliac limb; **c** right external iliac artery opened; left iliac limb filled with heparin; **d** repetition of outflow maneuvers in left iliac limb.

177

Closure of Retroperitoneum   The final maneuver is suturing the redundant aneurysm wall around the graft. This serves to assist in closing the retroperitoneal dead space and interposes a thick layer of tissue between the graft and the duodenum. Other than removing grossly degenerated and loosely attached fragments, it is not necessary to perform a complete endarterectomy of the aortic wall. Each iliac arm of the graft is wrapped separately to further obliterate dead space (**Fig. 6.22a–d**). The aneurysm wall

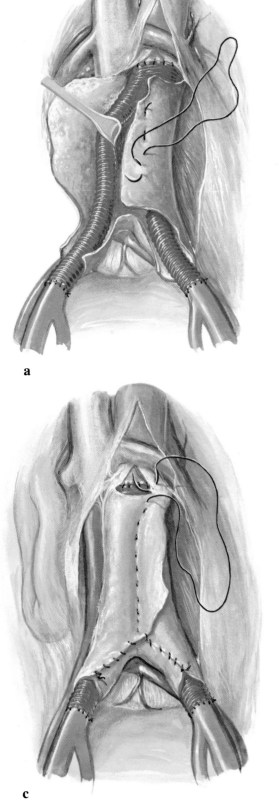

a

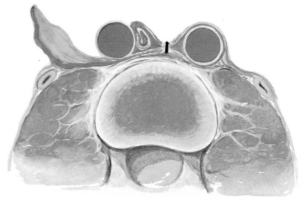

b

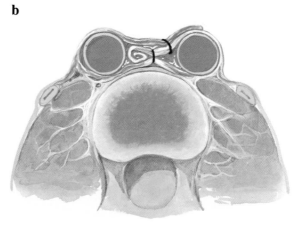

d

c

Fig. 6.22,a–d.   Coverage of graft with aneurysm wall. **a** closure over left iliac limb; **b** midline sutures to obliterate dead space; **c, d** overlapping flaps to further close dead space and extension of proximal sutures to include periaortic fibrous tissue in area of the proximal anastomosis.

178

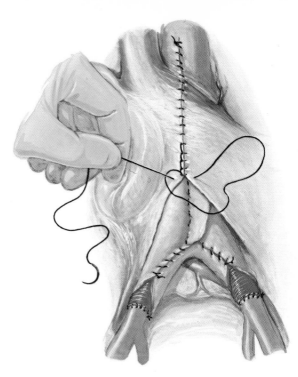

Fig. 6.23. Closure of posterior peritoneum to include wall of aneurysm.

rarely extends to a level that allows it to be used to cover the site of the proximal anastomosis. Coverage is thus accomplished by continuing the suture line proximally, utilizing the layer of periaortic fibrous tissue that was preserved at the time of skeletonizing the supra-aneurysmal aorta. Following this maneuver the graft, except for the distal iliac limbs, will be completely covered with tissue interposed between the graft and the duodenum. Approximation of the posterior peritoneum should utilize lock sutures to prevent telescoping of the duodenum (**Fig. 6.23**).

Variations

Posterior Adherence of Proximal Aorta Circumferential mobilization of the infrarenal aortic segment may occasionally be difficult to accomplish safely. If posterior finger dissection meets with resistance or threatens perforation of the aorta or dislodgment of friable intima, an alternate technique is illustrated in **Fig. 6.24a and b.** The posterior wall of the aorta is not transected. The posterior third of the graft anastomosis is made with deep sutures, which penetrate doubly the full thickness of the aortic wall.

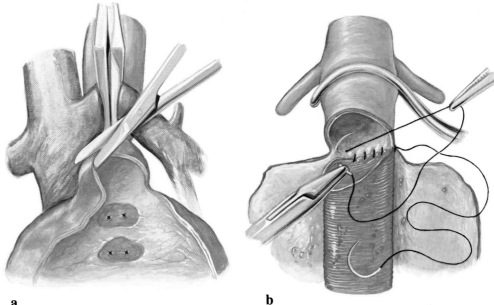

Fig. 6.24,a, b. Proximal anastomosis without posterior mobilization. **a** partial transection of aorta; **b** placement of posterior sutures.

a   b

179

Juxtorenal Origin of Aneurysm Occasionally the aneurysm begins so close to the renal arteries that it becomes impossible to apply safely an infrarenal clamp (**Fig. 6.25a**). In this situation it is often convenient to divide and suture the ends of the left renal vein to provide safe exposure for clamping of the suprarenal aorta (**Fig. 6.25b**). Preservation of the adrenal and gonadal branches of the vein provides adequate venous drainage for the left kidney and renal function is not compromised. One should reserve this maneuver until the final stage of the periaortic dissection, since the increased pressure in the left renal venous branches is conducive to profuse,

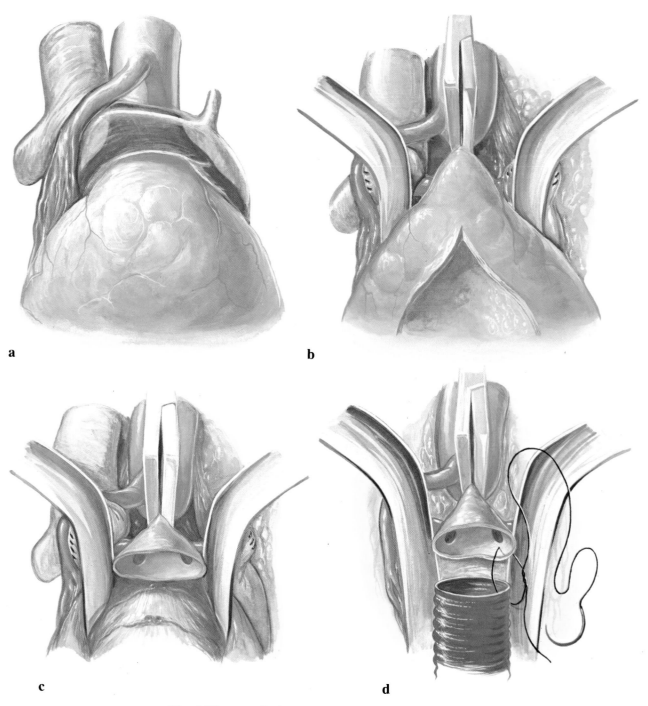

a

b

c

d

Fig. 6.25, a–d. Juxtarenal origin of aneurysm. **a** upper level of aneurysm at level of origin of renal arteries; **b** suprarenal aortic clamp in place; **c** level of aortic transection; **d** sutures placed adjacent to renal artery orifices.

difficult-to-control hemorrhage from retraction injuries. The aorta is transected subjacent to the renal arteries, preserving a cuff no longer than adequate to hold the anastomotic sutures (**Fig. 6.25c**). The sutures are placed in the aortic stump as close to the renal artery orifices as possible (**Fig. 6.25d**).

For infrarenal aneurysms that begin at the renal orifices, it is generally preferable to avoid transection or mobilization of the posterior wall of the aorta and to use the technique shown in Fig. 6.24. When enlargement of the aorta begins at this level, the media is assumed to have less than normal strength at this point. Each stitch in the posterior suture line will have passed through the full thickness of the aortic wall at two levels.

Distal Common Iliac Disease   Variations in performing the distal anastomoses often become necessary. The common iliac artery may be unacceptable for the customary end-to-end anastomosis because of aneurysmal dilatation extending to its bifurcation, or gross and extensive intimal disease at the same level (**Fig. 6.26a**).

This problem relates to the need for performing an operation that preserves forward flow into one or both hypogastric arteries. Terminal branches of the hypogastric artery connect with terminal branches of the IMA, and the hypogastric arteries thus become a source of collateral blood supply to the descending and sigmoid colon. If the IMA is not reimplanted into the aortic graft, loss of the hypogastric arteries could theoretically result in left colon ischemia, an event leading to early gangrene or late stricture of the bowel. In most patients the SMA, if patent, will provide adequate collateral flow to the left colon and the pelvis even with division of

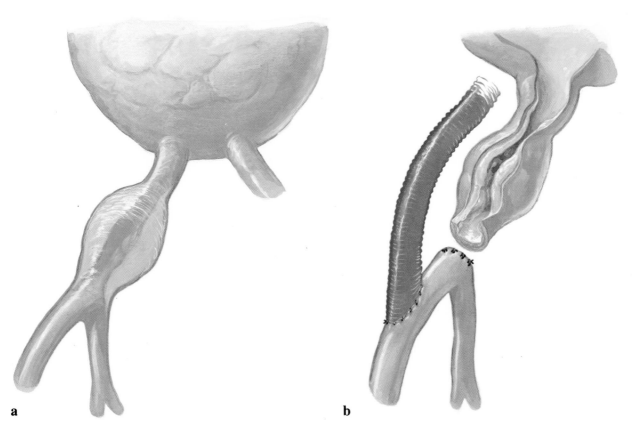

a   b

Fig. 6.26,a, b.   Distal extension of iliac disease. **a** advanced atheromatous lesion at iliac bifurcation; **b** graft to external iliac artery with preservation of common iliac stump.

the IMA (at its origin) and ligation of both hypogastric arteries. Preservation of the vessels in the sigmoid mesentery is essential to maintain this route of collateral flow to the colon.

The early stages of left colon ischemia involve the mucosa. Simple inspection of the color of the serosa may give the false impression that blood supply is adequate. A safer method is to evaluate the volume of backbleeding from the hypogastric arteries. If the backbleeding is profuse, these arteries may be safely ligated, and the iliac arms of the graft can be anastomosed end-to-end to the external arteries. If creating an end-to-end common iliac anastomosis is problematic on only one side, one can defer the decision of selecting the most appropriate reconstruction technique until after the opposite common iliac anastomosis has been completed and forward flow into that hypogastric artery established. Backbleeding from the hypogastric artery on the side in question will then usually be profuse, and simple unilateral hypogastric artery ligation can be performed without danger of compromising collateral flow.

Adequacy of blood flow to the left colon is also assured if vigorous backbleeding from the presewn stump of the IMA can be demonstrated. The orifice of this artery often will be occluded or severely stenosed and flow from the orifice may be scanty or absent, even with normal blood flow in its distal branches. For this reason, assessment of hypogastric blood flow is a more reliable determinant of decreased colon blood supply.

Even when adequate collateral flow to the pelvis has been demonstrated, preserving forward flow into the hypogastric arteries is preferable if at all feasible. If later resection of portions of the left colon should become necessary because of trauma, infection, or neoplasm, the collateral route to the more distal colon segment will be sacrificed.

One method for dealing with a troublesome common iliac artery is to extend the graft to the side of the external iliac artery (**Fig. 6.26b**). The common iliac stump is then oversewn, a maneuver that often must be preceded by the extraction of rigid intima adjacent to the end of the stump. Instrumental extraction of the intima in the stump in an attempt to provide a site for an end-to-end anastomosis to the common iliac artery is not recommended. An inadequate end point may become the cause of later thrombosis.

A dense periarterial inflammatory reaction surrounding the common iliac arteries often makes mobilizing them difficult without laceration of the iliac vein. In this circumstance, a safer maneuver is to oversew the iliac orifices from within the opened aorta (**Fig. 6.27**). Backbleeding can be controlled by clamps on the distal branches or by temporary insertion of balloon catheters into the iliac orifices until the closure has been nearly completed. The iliac graft arm can then be anastomosed to the side of either the common iliac or external iliac arteries.

Hypogastric Aneurysms Associated aneurysms of the hypogastric arteries are rare (**Fig. 6.28a**). When they do occur, the generalized aortoiliac lengthening forces them deep within the pelvis. The preoperative diagnosis is often made by the palpation of a pulsatile mass on rectal examination. Clamp control of their outflow arteries is frequently impossible to secure with safety. Even when control can be managed, suture of a graft deep in the pelvis is a formidable task. The safest means of management is simply to oversew the orifices of the outflow branches from within the aneurysm (**Fig. 6.28b and c**). If clamps cannot be applied distally, a finger on the outflow orifices controls bleeding while sutures are passed beneath it. An al-

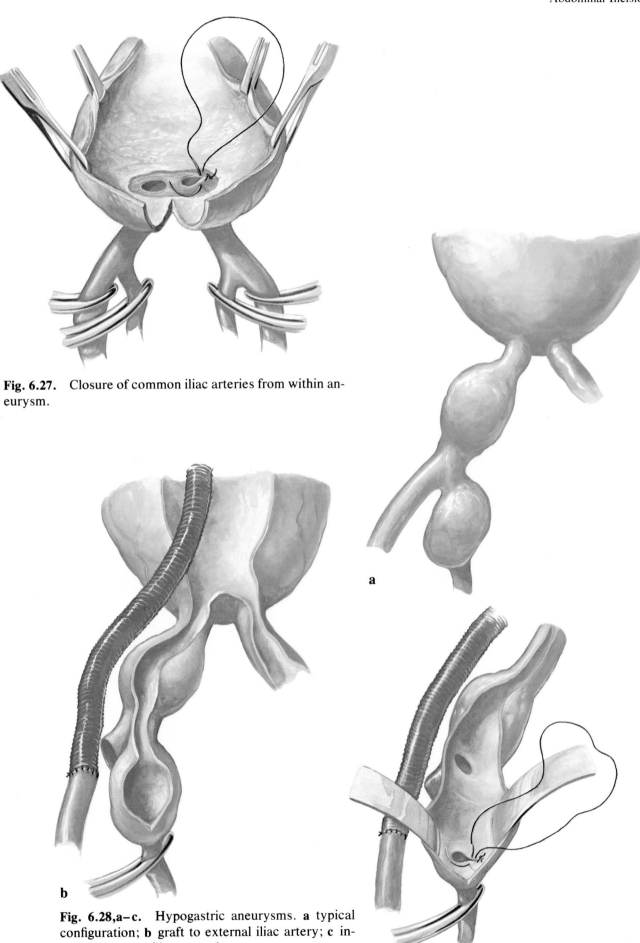

Fig. 6.27. Closure of common iliac arteries from within aneurysm.

a

b

Fig. 6.28,a–c. Hypogastric aneurysms. **a** typical configuration; **b** graft to external iliac artery; **c** internal closure of hypogastric artery.

c

183

ternate technique is to oversew the "neck" of the aneurysm at its origin. Blood pressure within the aneurysm will be low and the likelihood of subsequent rupture is remote. Either technique should be preceded by the hypogastric backflow evaluation described above.

Inflammatory Aneurysm   One unusual type of atherosclerotic aortic aneurysm has received scant attention in the literature and, for lack of a better word, has been called an "inflammatory" aneurysm (**Figs. 6.29–6.31**). The media, adventitia, and even the overlying anterior peritoneum become fused into a thick (2–3 cm) homogeneous layer with the rigidity of the rind of an unripened melon. The process begins on the anterior surface of the aneurysm and spreads laterally to involve as much as two-thirds of the aortic circumference. The "inflammatory" process tends to extend into the serosa of the duodenum or even the sigmoid colon if it falls against the aneurysm. The normal pinkness of the aneurysm surface is replaced by an ivory hue. Although the process is a sterile one, the term "inflammatory" aneurysm is appropriate because of the pain and tenderness that is produced. Symptoms may develop rapidly and often create the impression of a contained rupture of an aortic aneurysm. Although we have seen rupture of such an aneurysm in only one patient (the site of the rupture being in an

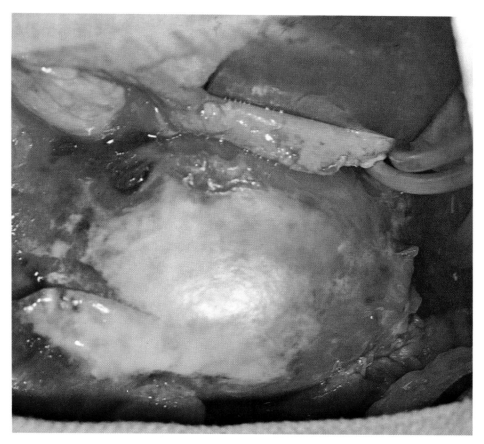

Fig. 6.29.   Presenting surface of an inflammatory atherosclerotic aneurysm of the infrarenal aorta. The latex tubing to the right encircles the left common iliac arteries. The patient's head is toward the left. The peritoneum is separable from the aneurysm only at its periphery. At top can be seen the peritoneal flap at the base of the sigmoid colon. The duodenum, visible at the lower left, is densely adherent to the aneurysm. The neck of the aneurysm (left) has been only partially mobilized at this stage.

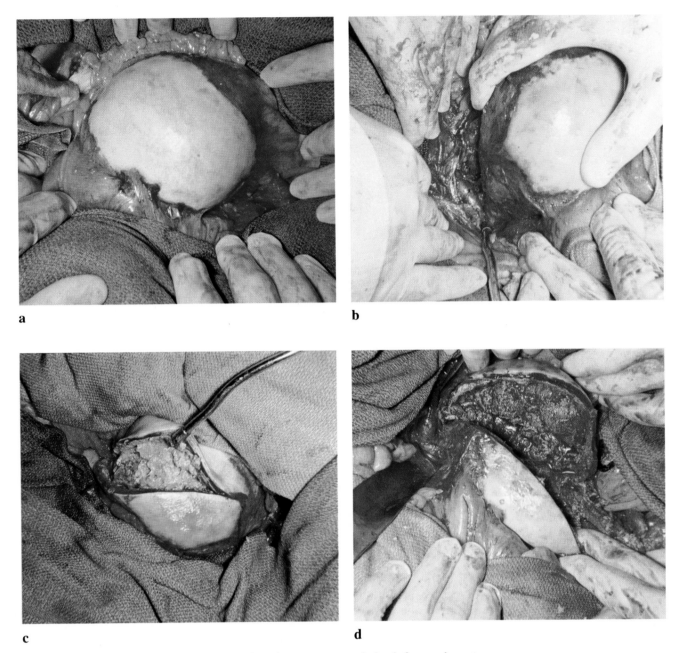

a

b

c

d

Fig. 6.30,a–d. Inflammatory atherosclerotic aneurysm of the infrarenal aorta. **a** As seen from the right side of the table before the dissection is started. The patient's head is to the left. Note the dense adherence of the duodenum below and the sigmoid mesentery above. **b** The proximal aorta and the left renal vein have been exposed (at the tip of the sucker). The duodenal attachment is preserved. **c** The initial incision of the aneurysm is through a thick wall that is almost cartilaginous in consistency. Note the layer of degenerated material in the aortic wall. **d** The circumferential mural thrombus that occupies most of the interior of the aneurysm has been evacuated. Note the granular thrombotic remnants attached to the inner surface. The duodenum remains attached to the rigid aortic wall.

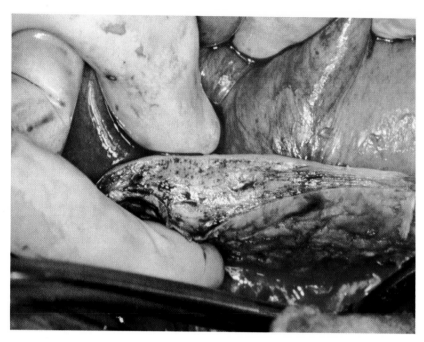

Fig. 6.31. Operative photograph of the rigid thick wall of an inflammatory aortic aneurysm held between the surgeon's thumb and forefinger. The attached duodenum can be seen in the upper right-hand corner.

uninvolved posterolateral surface of the aneurysm), many have been discovered at an emergency operation when the diagnosis of rupture could not be excluded.

At operation one finds that the process is confined to the distal two-thirds of the aneurysm, sparing the infrarenal aorta and the common iliac arteries. The usual dissection plane between the aorta and the duodenum is absent. An attempt to free the duodenum risks destroying its serosa, or entering its lumen before identifiable layers are seen, and therefore, it should be left attached to the aneurysm. The aneurysm is opened in the midline in the usual fashion (**Fig. 6.32a,b**). After removal of the contained thrombus, the wall remains rigid instead of collapsing as does the wall of the usual aneurysm. After the graft has been applied, the wall is folded over the prothesis with the duodenum still attached (**Fig. 6.32c**).

Preservation of Sexual Potency It appears at this time that a variation of the traditional operations for aortic aneurysms may be advisable in sexually active males. This recommendation stems from our observation that many males become impotent, in terms of their ability to obtain or maintain penile erection, after an otherwise satisfactory aneurysmectomy with graft replacement. In most of these, normal forward flow into both hypogastric arteries has been preserved. The most likely mechanism for this complication is transection of the preaortic plexus as it crosses the proximal left common iliac artery. This may occur during mobilization of the iliac arteries or as a result of extension of the aortotomy into them. This may be avoided by restricting mobilization of at least the left common iliac artery to its distal segment and leaving its proximal surface undisturbed. If local findings make an end-to-side anastomosis to the external iliac artery advisable, the orifice of the common iliac artery can be closed by internal sutures from within the aortotomy.

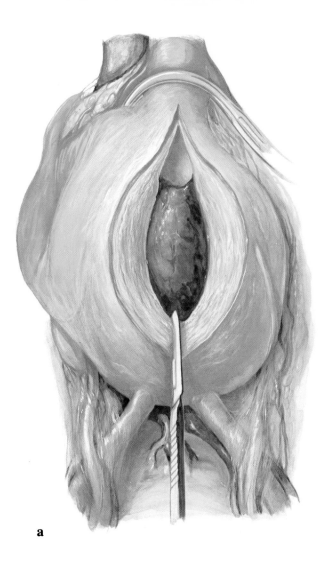

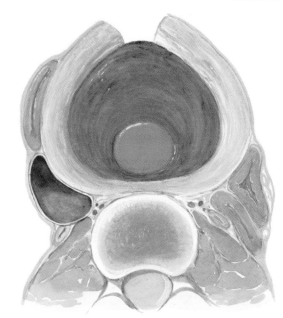

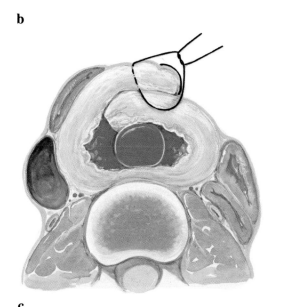

Fig. 6.32,a–c. Inflammatory aneurysm. **a** midline incision in aneurysm with duodenum undissected; **b** cross section of aneurysm after incision showing rigidity of its wall and the still-attached duodenum; **c** closure of aneurysm over graft.

Horseshoe Kidney The vascular surgeon's first encounter with a horseshoe kidney is often the result of a misdiagnosis. Laparotomy is performed after physical examination discloses a pulsatile midabdominal mass thought to be an aortic aneurysm in need of replacement. A normal aorta is found surrounded on both sides and across its front by a horseshoe kidney.

The reported frequency of horseshoe kidneys varied from 1 in 600–1800 individuals, and in 90% the kidneys are fused at the lower pole. The vascular pattern in most patients is similar to that in patients without a preaortic connection between the lower poles of the kidneys. Each half of the kidney is supplied by a single renal artery arising from the aorta at the usual position cephalad to the portion of the aorta in which the aortic aneurysm customarily develops. Anomalies in the vascular supply to the horseshoe kidney are more common, however, than in patients with normal kidneys and can be anticipated in slightly less than one-half of patients. These are the patients in whom special considerations will be required in the conduct of an operation to remove the aneurysm while maintaining adequate renal function.

187

As the presence of both an aortic aneurysm and a horseshoe kidney is rare, no single clinic can develop guidelines from its own experience that can deal with each of the numerous vascular anomalies. In most patients a preoperative intravenous urogram will provide the diagnosis of a horseshoe kidney, and an aortogram will ordinarily reveal anomalous renal arteries, if they are present, and suggest the most appropriate means for their management.

If a normal vascular pattern is identified, the isthmus usually may safely be divided in the midline, since frequently the connection between the lower poles is no more than a fibrous band. If the connection contains functioning parenchyma, the functioning ends should be oversewn. A useful method for determining the proper site for division is to clamp one of the renal arteries temporarily and observe the demarcation line between cyanosis and normal color in the isthmus. In some situations it is feasible to preserve the isthmus intact and tunnel the graft behind it.

If anomalous arteries are present, the three most common patterns of distribution are:

1. A single artery to each half of the kidney plus an additional artery to the isthmus.

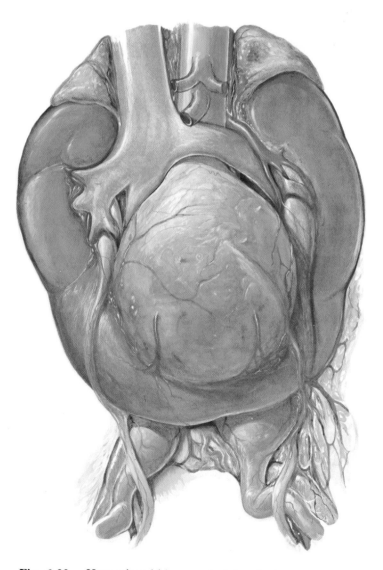

Fig. 6.33. Horseshoe kidney and abdominal aneurysm.

2. One or two renal arteries to each half and two arteries to the isthmus (Occasionally the inferior arteries arise from the common iliac arteries.)
3. Multiple renal arteries to all portions of the renal substance.

In the case of 1 or 2, the decision between resecting the portion of the kidney supplied by the extra renal arteries or reimplanting the lower arteries onto the graft to preserve renal mass (as illustrated in **Figs. 6.33 and 6.34**) depends in large part on the amount of renal parenchyma supplied by the additional arteries, which can be determined by observing the level of the line of demarcation following temporary occlusion of the respective arteries when the isthmic arteries arise from the aneurysm. Reimplantation will be unsuccessful in some situations since the disk-shaped section of the aorta that is removed with the artery will have a ragged, degenerated inner surface characteristic of the inner wall of an atherosclerotic aneurysm. In this situation, the risk of postoperative occlusion of the reimplanted artery would appear to be greater than if the aortic wall were normal.

When multiple renal arteries arise from all portions of the aneurysm to supply the bulk of the renal mass, the consequences of failure of multiple artery reimplantations becomes sizeable. In this situation, it may be well to reevaluate the indications for aneurysmectomy and to balance the morbidity of the unresected aneurysm against the possibility of renal failure with all that this implies in terms of chronic dialysis or renal transplantation.

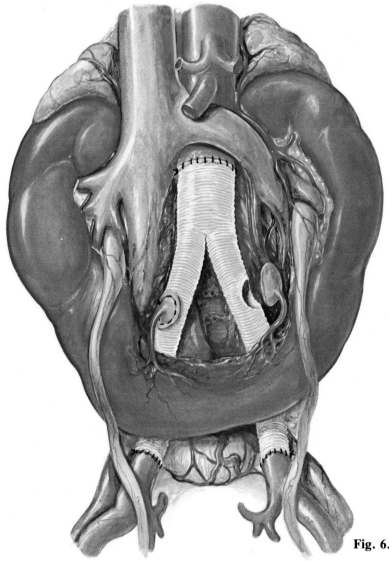

Fig. 6.34. Reimplantation of renal arteries in isthmus.

Suprarenal Abdominal Aortic Aneurysms

Patterns of Involvement

Aneurysmal disease of the suprarenal aorta may assume one of four patterns. The dumbbell shape shown in **Fig. 6.35a** is the most common. The infrarenal portion is usually the larger and often is the only portion requiring resection. If the diameter of the suprarenal component is less than 5 cm, the risk of rupture in this portion is generally less than the risk of removing the entire abdominal aorta. In this case, a conventional grafting operation is restricted to the infrarenal component of the aneurysm.

The next most common pattern is the generalized disease shown in **Fig. 6.35b.** Operation is indicated for rupture or when the maximum diameter exceeds 6–7 cm. The thoracic aorta, although cylindrically enlarged to some degree, has a wall of adequate strength for the proximal end of a grafting operation.

When the aneurysm is confined to the suprarenal aorta, it tends to be more globular than fusiform (**Fig. 6.35c**). The diagnosis is usually not suspected until symptoms appear. The most common presenting symptom is back pain from vertebral erosion. Operation is indicated for symptom relief, rupture, or in the asymptomatic good-risk patient, when the diameter of the aneurysm exceeds 6–7 cm.

A more extensive aneurysm is shown in **Fig. 6.35d**. It includes all or a large portion of the descending thoracic aorta, as well as most of the abdominal aorta. Because of the high mortality that accompanies aortic resection of this magnitude and the substantial frequency of postoperative paraplegia, the indications for operation are usually limited to intractable pain or excessive size of the aneurysm. If the patient is free of symptoms, operation is considered, if at all, only when aortic enlargement exceeds 9–11 cm.

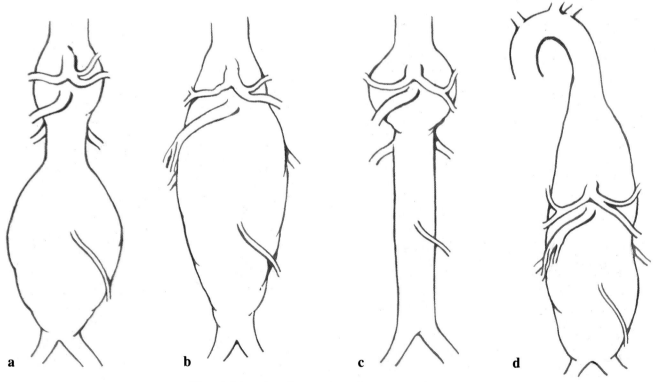

a   b   c   d

Fig. 6.35,a–d. Categories of suprarenal aneurysms. **a** dumbbell; **b** full-length abdominal; **c** suprarenal; **d** thoracoabdominal.

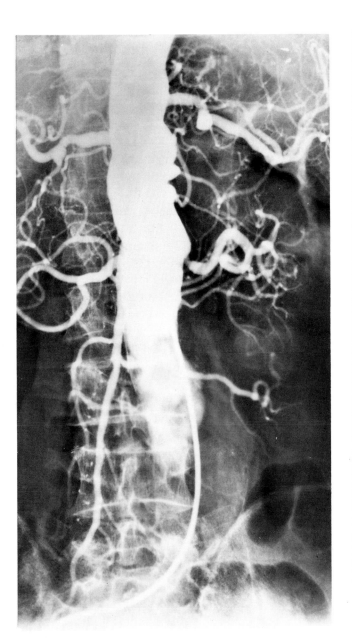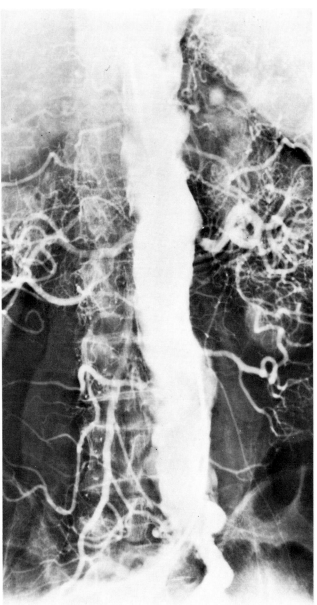

Fig. 6.35e. Sequential films from an aortogram in a 70-year-old patient with an infrarenal aortic aneurysm 8.5 cm in diameter. Renal function and blood pressure were normal. Mild dilatation of the thoracic aorta, revealed in a chest film, had suggested the possibility of a suprarenal component and the need for an aortogram. Note the 3-cm maximum diameter of the actual lumen of the infrarenal aorta. The remainder of the interior of the infrarenal aneurysm is occupied by the customary thick mural thrombus. Early aneurysmal degeneration has developed in the pararenal and suprarenal aortic segments. The irregular contour of the aortic lumen in this area suggests the presence of degenerated intima and/or mural thrombus. Moderate stenosis of the origin of the left renal artery is present.

The mild enlargement of the suprarenal aorta was not considered to be threatening and the left renal stenosis had not produced hypertension. For these reasons, operation was confined to replacement of the infrarenal aorta. The aortic clamp was placed cephalad to the celiac artery to avoid disruption of the intima in the suprarenal aortic segment.

The suprarenal portion of the aneurysm in any of the four patterns cannot be detected by abdominal palpation since it is proximal to the level of the xiphoid process. It is noteworthy that mild to moderate cylindrical enlargement of the thoracic aorta is almost uniformly present and is detectable by chest x-ray taken in the left anterior oblique projection. Thus, when dilatation of the thoracic aorta is demonstrated in a patient with a palpable infrarenal aneurysm, aortography by means of a catheter passed from the left axillary artery is advisable to determine the status of the suprarenal aorta. Sonography and computerized axial tomography have become valuable supplements in the diagnosis.

Thoracoabdominal Retroperitoneal Approach to the Aorta

Operations for abdominal aneurysms that involve the full length of the abdominal aorta or for the direct removal of atherosclerotic visceral artery lesions by transaortic endarterectomy (see Chapter 7) require an exposure that cannot be safely obtained by a simple abdominal incision. We have found that the thoracoabdominal retroperitoneal approach provides adequate exposure from the level of the distal thoracic aorta to the common iliac bifurcations. A retroperitoneal approach to the abdominal segment can be developed in a relatively avascular plane and lessens the visceral trauma of laparotomy.

The patient is placed in a supine position with sandbags under the left scapula. The subsequent torsion of the trunk tends to widen the incision and lessens the retraction requirements, while at the same time preserving access to the femoral arteries should reconstruction to this level become necessary. A left 8th-interspace thoracic incision is continued obliquely across the abdomen to beyond the midline. A retroperitoneal dissection plane is then developed that removes the peritoneum from the undersurface of the diaphragm and extends behind the spleen, pancreas, and intestines and anterior to the left kidney. The costochondral junction is transected and the pleura opened. A short segment of the cartilage is excised to avoid the discomfort of the frequent nonunion. The posterolateral fibers of the diaphragm are transected 3 cm from their costal origin by a circumferential incision that includes the thoracic pleura and posteriorly extends to the midline. This incision preserves the distal branches of the phrenic nerve and allows for earlier return of normal diaphragmatic function than if a radial muscle-splitting incision in the diaphragm were to be used. Transection of the inferior pulmonary ligament and the left crus of the diaphragm as it crosses the aorta provides exposure of the thoracic aorta to the T_9 level.

When this approach is used for patients requiring visceral artery revascularization, exposure of a lesser length of the thoracic aorta is required. Except for the left crus, the posterior 8–10 cm of the left hemidiaphragm can be left intact. The dense neural plexus surrounding the aorta at the level of the celiac and superior mesenteric arteries is divided and dissected free of the aorta. The visceral and renal arteries are skeletonized. The first branch of the SMA comes off its right side 6–7 cm from the aorta; thus, from this approach it is possible to mobilize the SMA without concern for encountering or damaging an important branch. **Fig. 6.36a–d** shows a patient at various stages of this approach.

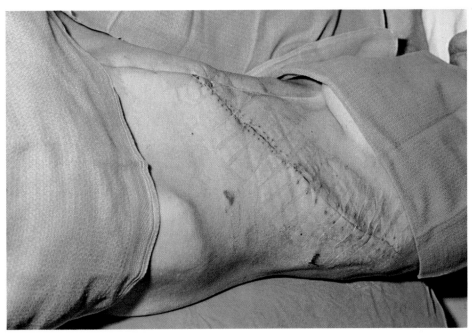

a

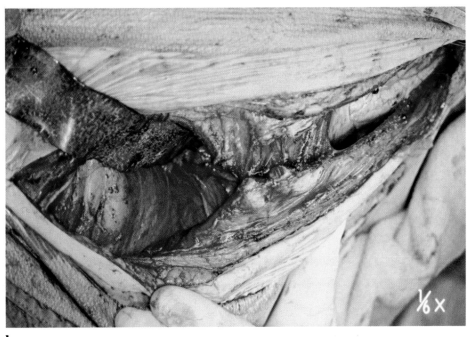

b

Fig. 6.36,a, b. Steps in the development of exposure in *thoracoretroperitoneal abdominal approach* to the aorta. (**b–d** taken from oblique angle to provide maximum visualization.) **a** The thoracic portion of the incision is placed in the 8th interspace and extended across the abdomen to the midline. If more distal exposure is required, incision is continued in the midline toward the symphysis pubis. At operation the patient is positioned with a greater degree of rotation of the trunk by elevation of the left scapula on sandbags.

b The peritoneum in the left flank and on the undersurface of the diaphragm has been dissected free in a maneuver that will eventually allow the encased peritoneal contents to be dislocated across the midline, leaving the kidney and adrenal gland behind. The pleural space has been entered to the right. The costal cartilage is still intact. Note the left lower lobe of the lung and the superior surface of the diaphragm to the right.

193

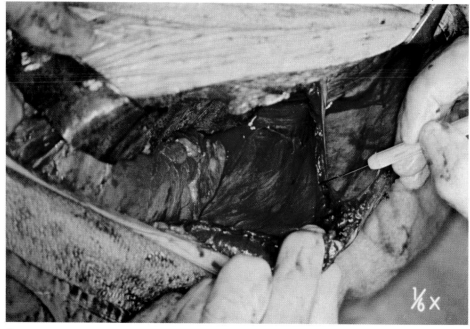

c

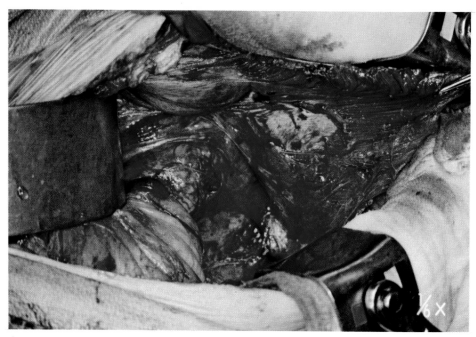

d

Fig. 6.36,c, d. **c** The costal cartilage has been cut and a short segment removed. The diaphragm, with its attached pleural lining, is cut circumferentially adjacent to the origin of its fibers.

d The most posterior fibers of the diaphragm are left intact. The fibers covering the aorta have been transected. Further proximal exposure of the aorta is obtained by splitting the fibers to the right on its surface. The posterior surface of the spleen (top) is behind the intact peritoneum.

Replacement Graft with Transposition of Visceral Branches

Fig. 6.37a–h shows the successive steps in a grafting operation in patients with aneurysms illustrated in Fig. 6.35b,c,d. **Fig. 6.38a and b** shows pre- and postoperative photographs of a similar operation. There are several

Fig. 6.37,a–h. Graft replacement of full-length abdominal aneurysm.

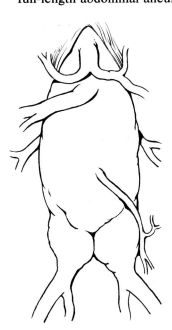

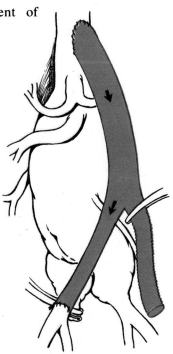

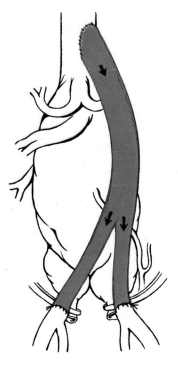

a extent of aneurysm

b bypass graft with right iliac anastomosis completed

c left iliac anastomosis

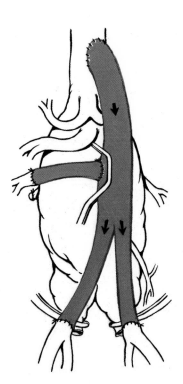

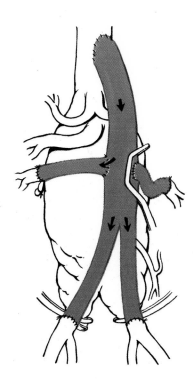

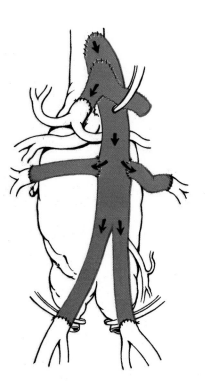

d graft to right renal artery

e left renal graft in place

f small bifurcated cephalad side arm with one limb to celiac artery

195

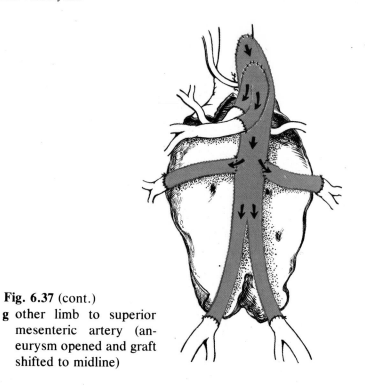

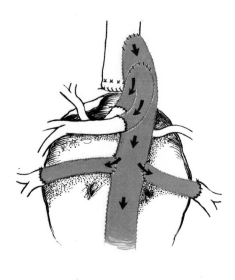

Fig. 6.37 (cont.)
g other limb to superior mesenteric artery (aneurysm opened and graft shifted to midline)

h proximal aorta transected and oversewn

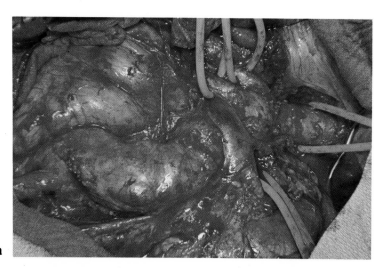

a

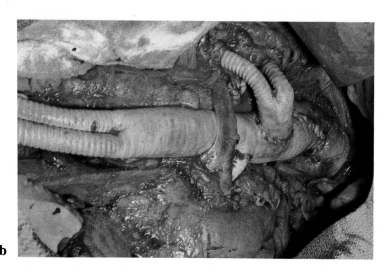

Fig. 6.38,a, b. Operative photographs (**a**) before and (**b**) after graft replacement of an atherosclerotic aneurysm involving the full length of the abdominal aorta. The aortic graft has been anastomosed to the side of the distal thoracic aorta and side arms extended to the celiac and superior mesenteric arteries by way of a small (10 × 5-mm) bifurcation graft. The renal arteries have individual side-arm grafts and the distal iliac grafts have end-to-end anastomoses to the common iliac arteries. The distal thoracic aorta has been transected and closed as the final maneuver before resection of the aneurysm. A thoracoabdominal approach has been used.

b

equally suitable modifications of this technique; the basic principle in all of them is the preservation of blood flow within the aneurysm until its four major branches have been individually transferred to the aortic portion of the functioning prosthesis. With the technique shown, forward flow in the aneurysm has been preserved until all the anastomoses have been completed. An alternate technique in patients with this type of aneurysm would be one in which the iliac arms of the graft were anastomosed end-to-side to the patient's iliac arteries as the first step. An end-to-end anastomosis of the prosthesis to the aorta proximal to the aneurysm would then produce retrograde flow from the iliac arteries into the distal aorta and its visceral and renal branches while the individual branches were transferred to the prosthesis.

Replacement Graft with Intraluminal Anastomoses of Visceral Branches

Dr. Stanley Crawford has introduced another technique shown in **Fig. 6.39a–e.** The aneurysm is opened widely as the first step. The anastomosis between the proximal aorta and the prosthesis is established, followed in rapid succession by suture of the aortic wall adjacent to each of the four major branches to generous openings at appropriate positions on the graft. An experienced surgeon should encounter little difficulty in restoring normal renal blood within the tolerance time of renal ischemia. The drawings in this series indicate that a periorifice endarterectomy has been performed to deal with stenosis of the right renal artery. The suture line in all of the

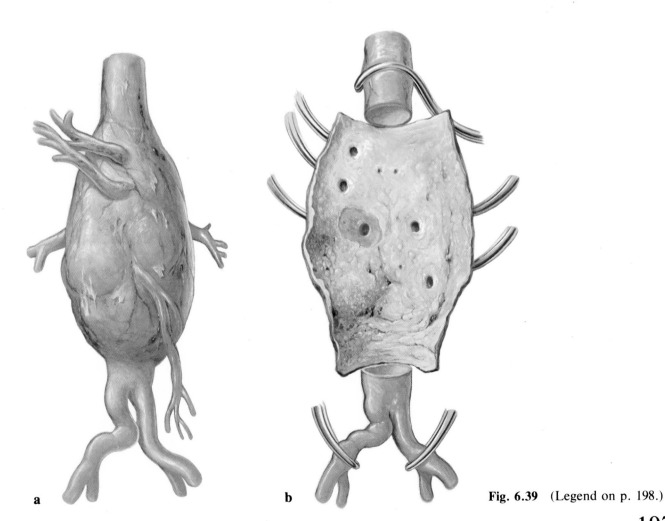

a   b   **Fig. 6.39**   (Legend on p. 198.)

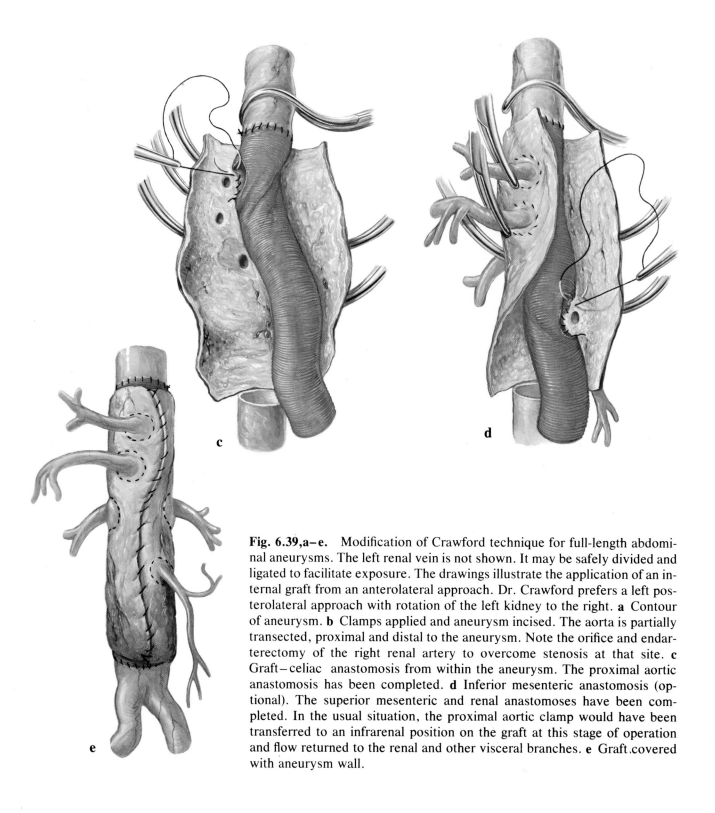

Fig. 6.39,a–e. Modification of Crawford technique for full-length abdominal aneurysms. The left renal vein is not shown. It may be safely divided and ligated to facilitate exposure. The drawings illustrate the application of an internal graft from an anterolateral approach. Dr. Crawford prefers a left posterolateral approach with rotation of the left kidney to the right. **a** Contour of aneurysm. **b** Clamps applied and aneurysm incised. The aorta is partially transected, proximal and distal to the aneurysm. Note the orifice and endarterectomy of the right renal artery to overcome stenosis at that site. **c** Graft–celiac anastomosis from within the aneurysm. The proximal aortic anastomosis has been completed. **d** Inferior mesenteric anastomosis (optional). The superior mesenteric and renal anastomoses have been completed. In the usual situation, the proximal aortic clamp would have been transferred to an infrarenal position on the graft at this stage of operation and flow returned to the renal and other visceral branches. **e** Graft covered with aneurysm wall.

aorta–branch artery anastomoses is sufficiently removed from each orifice so that intimal fragmentation at the site of the sutures would not compromise the arterial orifice.

The major advantages of this technique over the one previously described are the reduction of the number of anastomoses and the elimination of anastomoses between small grafts and small arteries. For the extensive aneurysms illustrated in Fig. 6.35d, blood supply to the spinal cord is preserved by including the intercostal and the proximal lumbar arteries in the intra-aneurysmal anastomoses. This is probably the only technique that is applicable when rupture of the suprarenal segment of the aneurysm—shown in Fig. 6.35a or in any portion of the aneurysm as shown in Fig. 6.35b–d—has occurred.

Ruptured Abdominal Aneurysm

Rupture of an atherosclerotic aneurysm of the abdominal aorta is the result of gradual disintegration of the media until it can no longer resist the blood pressure within the lumen. Although rupture can occur at any stage of development, it most commonly occurs after the aortic diameter exceeds 6 cm. The first event is usually rupture into the space between the adventitia and the periaortic fibrous tissue accompanied by pain and a transient fall in systemic blood pressure. The periaortic hematoma is contained in this plane as long as tissue strength exceeds the reduced intra-aortic pressure. Blood loss is minimal and systemic pressure rapidly returns to normal. The rupture may remain contained for periods varying from an hour to several days. This is the golden period for surgical intervention before prolonged shock and resulting multiorgan damage has occurred from progression to the next phase. The second stage develops when blood breaks through its new capsule and flows into the retroperitoneal space. The patient now presents in frank shock and with each added minute the potential for survival, even after a technically successful operation, lessens.

Shock
When acute abdominal pain and/or acute fall of blood pressure occurs in the presence of a palpable pulsatile abdominal mass, the diagnosis is rupture of an abdominal aneurysm unless proved otherwise. The only reliable proof is obtained by *immediate* laparotomy and *nothing* should delay its performance. Mortality involved in an operation performed before shock has developed can be negligible. When shock is present, the mortality rate approaches 75%. A fall in blood pressure should be corrected by rapid volume replacement during the preparation for, and the beginning of, operation.

The first operative maneuver, which takes precedence over all others, is the control of hemorrhage, and in so doing, one may need to forego all the niceties of preparation for an elective operation, e.g., shaving the abdomen, a 10-minute scrub, etc. It is important to recognize that the induction of anesthesia may abolish the normal vasoconstrictive responses that have maintained blood pressure during the period of increasing hypovolemia. Wide-bore venous catheters should be inserted as early as possible to permit massive blood replacement during the induction of anesthesia.

Operative Technique
At laparotomy the appearance of a contained rupture is usually little more than a discolored bulge under the peritoneum over a portion of the anterolateral aspect of the aneurysm proximal to the level of the inferior mesenteric artery. If the patient's blood pressure remains stable at a normal level, the iliac arteries should be mobilized and prepared for grafting before the proximal aorta is approached. The proximal dissection may unroof the site of rupture and desirably all should be in readiness for the definitive operation.

199

If the rupture is no longer contained, the entire retroperitoneum will be discolored and projected forward, obscuring the actual contour of the aneurysm (**Fig. 6.40a**). In this situation, the first move should be to control the bleeding by proximal occlusion of the aorta. The hematoma will usually have created the periaortic dissection plane by encircling the aorta at the proximal end of the aneurysm. After the posterior peritoneum has been incised, the surgeon's finger is thrust into the hematoma and advanced along the superior surface of the aneurysm until the normal infrarenal aorta is reached (**Fig. 6.40b**). The finger is then inserted posteriorly on each side of the aorta to the level of the vertebral bodies (**Fig. 6.41a–c**).

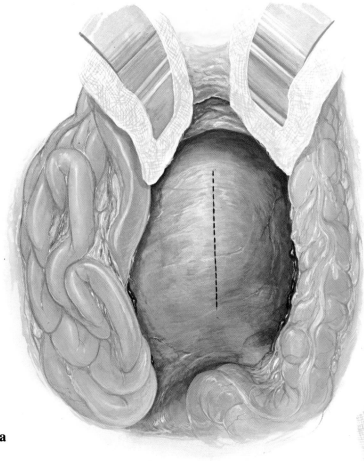

a

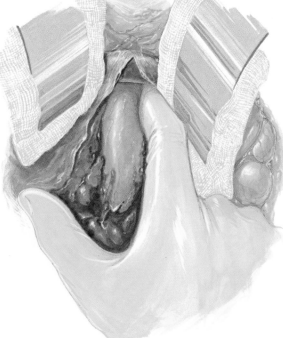

b

Fig. 6.40,a, b. Approach to proximal aorta. **a** retroperitoneal hematoma; **b** finger dissection within hematoma.

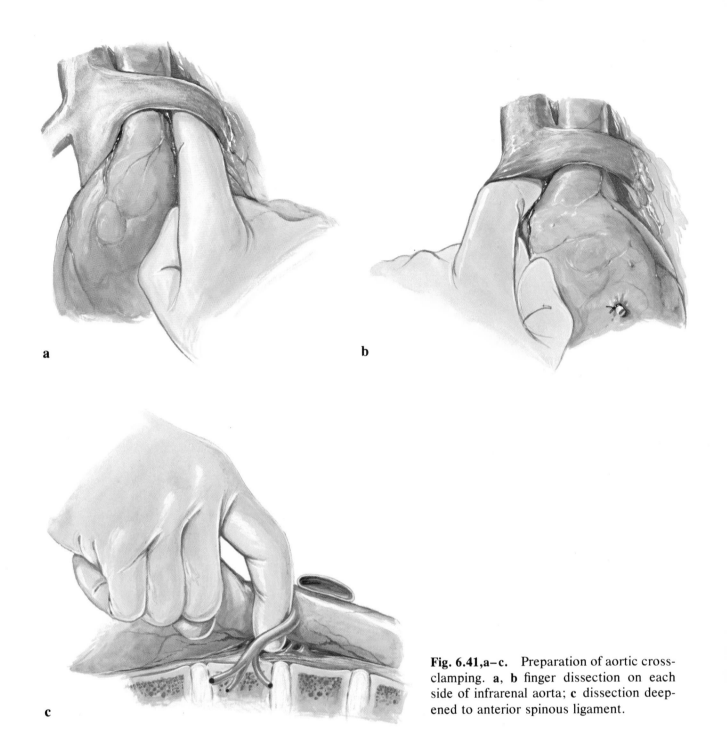

a

b

c

Fig. 6.41,a–c. Preparation of aortic cross-clamping. **a, b** finger dissection on each side of infrarenal aorta; **c** dissection deepened to anterior spinous ligament.

With the finger still in place on the right side of the aorta to displace the inferior vena cava, the opened jaws of an aortic clamp are inserted on each side of the aorta and closed. It is important that both the dissecting finger and the clamp approach the aorta at the beginning of the aneurysmal bulge. Since these maneuvers are performed blindly, a more cephalad approach risks laceration of the left renal vein. If the renal vein is inadvertently torn, it should be immediately crossclamped and divided.

Once the aorta has been clamped and hemorrhage arrested, the continuation of blood replacement usually promptly restores systemic blood pressure to normal levels. While this is occurring, further dissection to develop an adequate proximal aortic stump can be carried out in an orderly way.

201

If the finger dissection described above dislodges a clot from the site of rupture, the operative field is immediately obscured by the gush of fresh blood. Should this occur, the aneurysm should immediately be incised to permit insertion of the surgeon's thumb into the infrarenal aorta (**Fig. 6.42**). The neck of the aneurysm is almost always smaller than the first or second joint of the thumb. With the thumb in place, the remainder of the aneurysm can be unroofed and balloon catheters passed into the common iliac orifices to control backbleeding (**Fig. 6.43**).

At this stage one of two maneuvers can be performed. The supraceliac aorta can be either mobilized for crossclamping or simply occluded by compression with a concave plunger (**Fig. 6.44**). The alternate technique is to insert a 30-ml Foley catheter into the proximal aorta along the side of the occluding thumb (**Fig. 6.45a**). Inflation of the balloon controls the proximal aorta and allows removal of the thumb (**Fig. 6.45b**). The catheter should previously be threaded through the graft so that, if necessary, it remains in place until the proximal anastomosis has been completed (**Fig. 6.45c**). In the more usual situation, it is possible to mobilize the normal infrarenal aorta at this time to permit removal of the balloon and application of a clamp across the aorta below the renal arteries.

Variations

Two other types of aortic rupture deserve special mention because of the different manner of their presentation. In one, the rupture occurs on the left posterolateral aspect and blood dissects into a plane behind the psoas

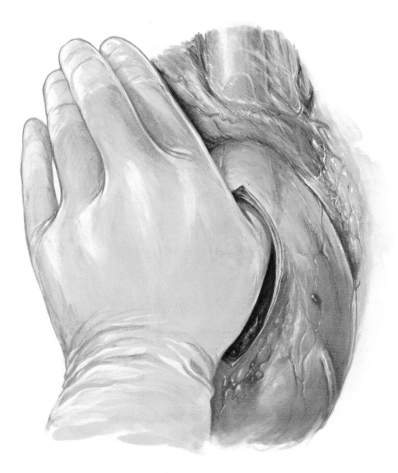

Fig. 6.42. Insertion of thumb into proximal aorta for emergency control.

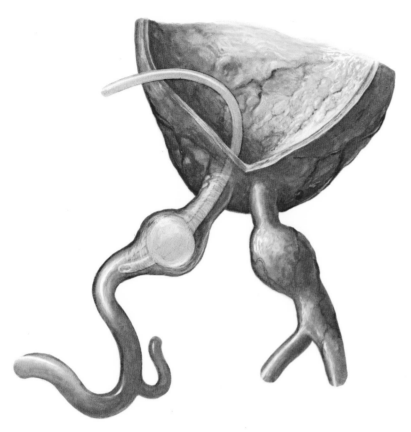

Fig. 6.43. Internal balloon catheter control of common iliac arteries.

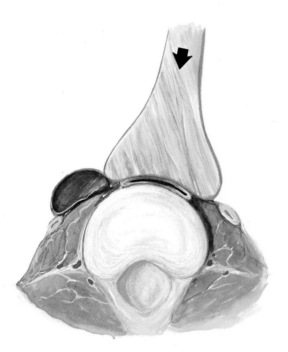

Fig. 6.44. Supraceliac aortic compression. The original wood external aortic occluder fashioned for this purpose has now been replaced with a commercially available metal one.

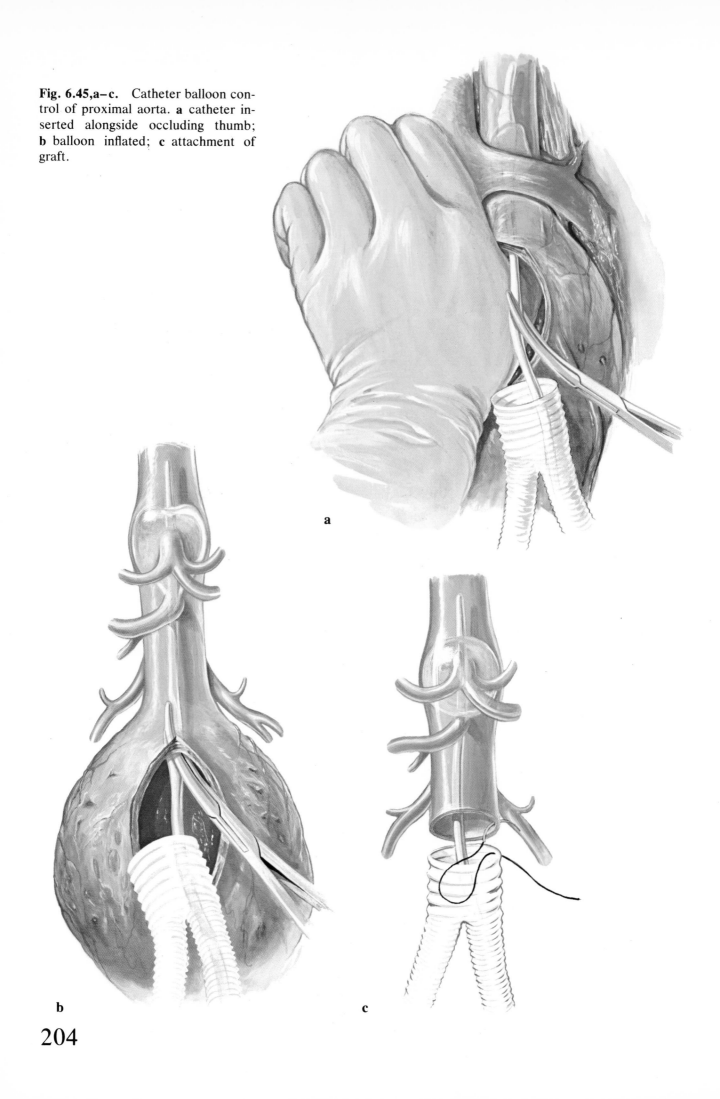

Fig. 6.45, a–c. Catheter balloon control of proximal aorta. **a** catheter inserted alongside occluding thumb; **b** balloon inflated; **c** attachment of graft.

a

b

c

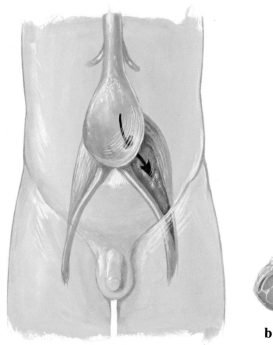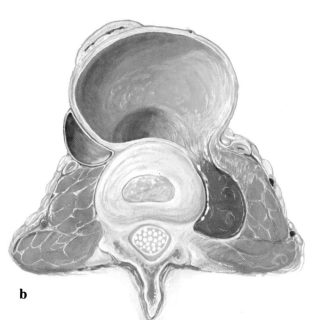

a   b

Fig. 6.46,a, b. Parapsoas dissection.

muscle (**Fig. 6.46a and b**). It then follows the course of a psoas abscess toward and even into the groin. The time of containment in this cavity is generally longer than the containment period of the usual form of rupture. The patient complains of severe left lower-quadrant pain. He will lie with the thigh flexed, and attempts to straighten the thigh intensifies the pain. In the patients we have seen, the rupture is usually at the site of a bleb in a relatively small aortic aneurysm (<5 cm in diameter). The diagnosis is suspected by the palpation of a tender pulsatile fullness in the left lower quadrant and a positive psoas sign. Operative management is the same as for an elective aneurysmectomy.

The other unusual presentation occurs from rupture of a bleb on the right side of what is usually also a small aneurysm. In this case the rupture breaks into the wall of the vena cava, creating a massive arteriovenous fistula. The presenting picture is usually one of acute congestive heart failure in a patient with a widened pulse pressure. A loud abdominal machinery murmur is usually present. Abdominal pain and tenderness are less than in the usual form of rupture. The diagnosis should be suspected in any patient with acute cardiac failure with any combination of findings of abdominal pain, an enlarged aorta, or an abdominal bruit with a wide pulse pressure. Immediate closure of the fistula is mandatory to prevent death from cardiac failure.

At operation, immediate crossclamping of the infrarenal aorta, the iliac arteries, and the inferior mesenteric artery should be the first maneuvers. The aorta is then incised longitudinally. The orifice of the fistula will be identified by the venous bleeding. The opening is usually smaller than a fingertip and bleeding is arrested by finger compression. A larger opening can be controlled by insertion of two balloon catheters into the opening to occlude the proximal and distal vena cava. Prior mobilization of the inferior vena cava is unnecessary and time consuming. The opening is closed by deep transverse sutures that include in one layer the walls of the aorta and the vena cava. Normal continuity should not be impaired. The remainder of the operation is performed as with an elective aneurysmectomy.

Visceral Atherosclerosis

7

Atherosclerotic stenosis or occlusion of the celiac and superior mesenteric arteries is the most common cause of the unique syndrome of chronic visceral ischemia. The characteristic pattern of postprandial epigastric pain, reluctance to eat, and resultant and usually profound weight loss is not duplicated by any other disease. Atherosclerosis in this location is encountered more frequently in females than males and often in the midadult years. Because this sex–age combination is an unusual one in patients with atherosclerosis at other sites, the diagnosis of visceral atherosclerosis is often overlooked in the initial evaluation.

The visceral artery lesions are usually associated with a unique variant of atherosclerosis in which the entire abdominal aorta develops a homogeneous succulent layer of intimal thickening that virtually overflows the orifices of the visceral arteries. Not uncommonly the renal arteries become involved as well. In the celiac artery, the atherosclerotic lesion is confined to the first half of this relatively short artery. Even when celiac stenosis progresses to occlusion, the distal undiseased half of the artery retains its patency due to the high volume of interconnecting collateral flow in its three terminal branches.

Superior mesenteric artery occlusion is a more lengthy lesion. When atheroma occludes its orifice, the static column of blood distal to it clots to the level of the first major branch that is returning collateral flow to the distal branches. The result is an occluded segment usually 5–8 cm in length. The short lesion in celiac occlusion is easily removed by a simple transaortic endarterectomy; the more lengthy lesion in SMA occlusion requires a supplementary angioplasty. It is important to note that the advanced form of aortic disease noted above is confined to the abdominal portion of the aorta. The thoracic aorta is only minimally involved, a finding of practical significance in the design of a durable revascularization technique. Twenty percent of patients will have substantial atherosclerotic disease in the infrarenal abdominal aorta, either occlusive or aneurysmal, which must be dealt with when operation is indicated for visceral ischemic symptoms.

Aortography is the only study that provides a definitive diagnosis. This study should preferably be obtained by the Seldinger catheter technique with AP, cross table lateral and occasionally oblique views to delineate the arterial orifices and patterns of collateral flow. When either the su-

207

perior mesenteric or the celiac artery become sufficiently narrowed to impair blood flow, collateral channels in the gastroduodenal pancreatico-duodenal connections will become apparent. SMA occlusion also stimulates visible collateral flow from the inferior mesenteric artery by way of the "meandering mesenteric" artery. When all three visceral branches of the aorta are occluded, collateral flow may ascend into the abdomen from one or both hypogastric arteries. These large collateral channels are often adequate to maintain adequate visceral circulation when one or more of the visceral arteries are occluded. Thus, the radiologic demonstration of visceral artery occlusion and collateral channels are not in themselves indications for surgical intervention.

Considerable debate exists regarding the number and location of obstructive lesions that must be present to produce symptoms of chronic visceral ischemia. The most frequently expressed opinion is that at least two of the visceral branches of the aorta must be obstructed. Our own observations support this in part, but suggest that symptoms are related more to the inadequacy of collateral blood flow than to the actual number of obstructed primary arteries. This opinion is based on clinical observations of four categories of patients: (1) those with one or more visceral artery lesions without visceral ischemic symptoms (aortography performed for other reasons); (2) symptomatic patients with one or more visceral artery occlusions; (3) patients with multiple visceral artery involvement in whom an operation was performed on only one artery; and (4) symptomatic patients in whom the superior mesenteric and celiac arteries were repaired but in whom postoperative occlusion of one artery was revealed by the follow-up aortogram.

These have led to the following conclusions:

1. Most symptomatic patients have occlusion or stenosis of more than one of the three visceral branches of the aorta.
2. An occasional asymptomatic patient will have occlusion of two or even all three of these branches.
3. Chronic orifice lesions that involve the SMA or the IMA alone rarely produce symptoms.
4. An orifice lesion in the celiac artery is the only one in which a single chronic visceral artery lesion may produce symptoms.

These observations and the pathologic considerations noted above have led to the adoption of certain principles in determining the need for a reconstructive vascular operation and in the selection of the most appropriate approach.

1. Occlusion or stenosis of one or more visceral arteries is generally not an indication for operation unless symptoms of chronic visceral ischemia are present.
2. A revascularization operation is indicated in any patient with the characteristic pain syndrome of chronic visceral ischemia when atherosclerotic lesions involve one or more visceral branches. In this case the objectives are twofold: one, to relieve pain; two, to prevent visceral infarction as the disease progresses.
3. The ideal operation is one that provides normal blood flow to all three visceral branches of the aorta. It is acknowledged that a residual single SMA or IMA occlusion is ordinarily well tolerated because of the usual availability of collateral flow from proximal or distal arteries. However, should the patient later require a resection operation for gastroduodenal or left colon disease, it may be necessary to sacrifice these collateral channels.

4. If a complete operation is not feasible, the priorities for revascularization, in order of importance, are the celiac, the SMA, and the IMA. In an elective operation on a poor-risk patient or an urgent operation for early or impending intestinal infarction in patients with chronic celiac and SMA occlusions, restoration of celiac patency alone can be expected to restore intestinal viability and function.

5. For grafting operations the ideal alignment of the graft is one that courses antegrade and parallel to both the parent and recipient arteries in order to minimize turbulence and lessen the potential for graft occlusion. The appropriate point of origin of such a graft should be in an undiseased segment that is not susceptible to the later development of obstructive atherosclerosis either at the site of anastomosis or proximal to it. These conditions are met in visceral grafting operations only when the graft originates from the distal thoracic aorta. We have largely avoided grafts that originate from the infrarenal aorta because of the reversal of flow direction (usually at both ends) and the vulnerability of the aorta at this level to the later development of obstructive atherosclerosis.

6. When endarterectomy is to be used, the approach and technique should be one that provides safe access to and exposure of the entire abdominal aorta in order to permit the surgeon to carry out a definitive procedure in all visceral branches and to manage associated and infrarenal aortic lesions if they are present.

Bypass Grafts

To meet the conditions for bypass grafts described in No. 5 above, we have used grafts from the distal thoracic aorta in the form of either simple grafts to the celiac artery or bifurcation grafts to both the celiac artery and the SMA. Either operation may be performed through an abdominal approach.

A tubular graft extending from the anterior surface of the aorta at the T_{10} level to the distal end of the transected celiac artery in patients with combined celiac and SMA disease has proved to be an effective operation for augmenting total visceral blood flow. In most patients there are large communications between the terminal branches of the celiac artery and the superior mesenteric artery; thus, a residual occlusion of the proximal SMA is well tolerated. This operation is potentially less effective in patients with associated occlusion of the IMA or in the case of the rare anomaly of a superior mesenteric origin of the common hepatic artery. Its effect may be nullified if a later intestinal operation destroys the collateral pathways. In patients with combined celiac and SMA lesions, we have used the grafting operation to the celiac artery only for those whose poor general condition made the more extensive operation of transaortic endarterectomy or the implantation of a bifurcation graft to both arteries too hazardous to undertake.

The preferred graft material has been knitted Dacron. Of the 10 that have been used, all have remained patent. We have abandoned saphenous vein grafts in this position because of the high frequency of late closure (5 out of 6 in our experience). In none of the patients in which synthetic grafts have been implanted has bowel necrosis or peritoneal sepsis been present.

The approach to the celiac artery and the supraceliac aorta is through the gastrohepatic ligament. Reflection of the left lobe of the liver to the right and retraction of the esophagus to the left exposes the posterior fibers of the diaphragm. Separation of these fibers in the midline provides a retropleural exposure of the distal thoracic aorta (**Fig. 7.1**).

After proximal and distal crossclamping, an elliptical aortotomy is made on the anterior surface of the supraceliac aorta (**Fig. 7.2a and b**). A 5 or 6 mm Dacron graft cut from a 10 × 5 or 12 × 6 bifurcation graft to provide a flange for the proximal end is anastomosed to the aortotomy (**Fig. 7.2c**). The aortic clamps are then released. The period of aortic occlusion rarely exceeds 5 min. The distal end of the graft is anastomosed end-to-end to the celiac artery that has been transected distal to the diseased segment at the celiac orifice.

Our experience with bifurcation grafts from the thoracic aorta to both the celiac artery and the SMA in patients with combined disease is more recent, but the early results have been encouraging. Thus far, its use has been limited to patients whose stenotic lesions had not progressed to total occlusion. In this situation the two arteries retain a lumen of normal size beyond the proximal orifice lesions and are available for simple end-to-end anastomoses to the respective limbs of the bifurcated graft. Total occlusion at the celiac orifice, however, does not create a contraindication for an end-to-end anastomosis since the distal half of the celiac artery

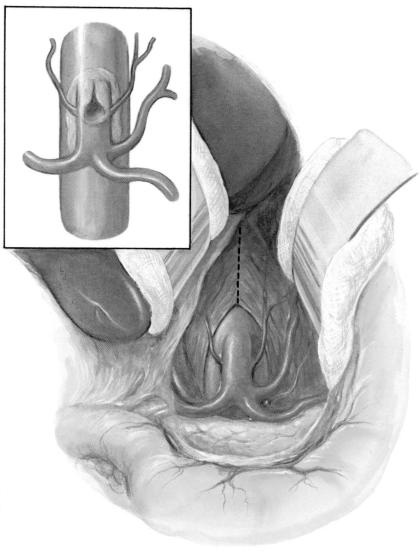

Fig. 7.1. Anterior approach to celiac artery and supraceliac aorta. **Inset** distribution of a typical celiac atherosclerotic lesion with adjacent aortic extension.

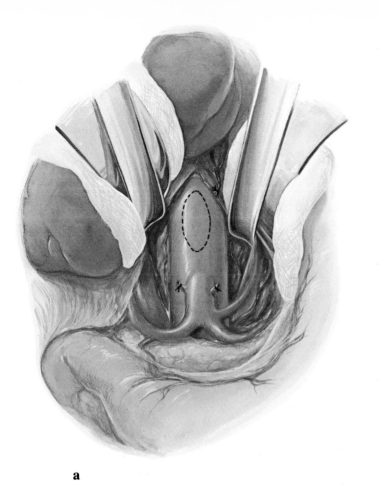

a

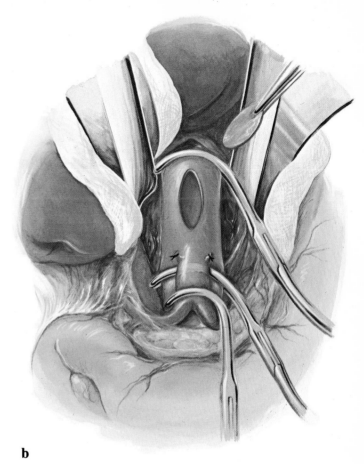

b

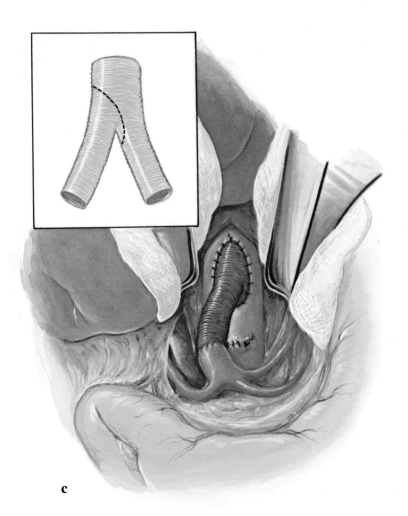

c

Fig. 7.2, a–c. Aortoceliac graft. **a** position of aortotomy; **b** celiac artery prepared for transection; **c** completed graft. **Inset** Note the flange on the graft prepared by cutting it from a bifurcated graft.

211

usually remains patent. Total occlusion at the SMA orifice is a more lengthy lesion, and an end-to-side anastomosis would be more appropriate if a limb of the graft were to be extended to the SMA.

The route of entry to the region of the terminal thoracic aorta and to the origins of the celiac artery and the SMA is the same as the one used for aorta–celiac bypass. Incision in the posterior peritoneum caudad to the base of the transverse mesocolon is not required. After division and separation of the pre-aortic fibers of the diaphragm, resection of the neural plexus surrounding the celiac artery and overlying the aorta caudad to it exposes the origins of both arteries and frees the body of the pancreas from its posterior attachments (**Figs. 7.3–7.5**). Caudad retraction of the body of the pancreas provides exposure for easy mobilization of the first 4–5 cm of the SMA.

Fig. 7.6 shows the position of the aortotomy and line of transection of the exposed celiac and SMA. An oblique elliptical anterolateral aortotomy for the proximal anastomosis allows the left limb of the graft to course anterior to the aorta for its union with the transected end of the celiac artery. The right limb extends along the right anterolateral aspect of the aorta and behind the pancreas to a position alongside and parallel to the course of the SMA, thereby permitting an "in-line" graft to artery anastomosis (**Figs. 7.7–7.9**). The dimensions of a 12 × 6 mm knitted bifurcation graft are appropriate in most circumstances.

The advantages of the two grafting technics described are the absence of disease in the parent artery (the thoracic aorta), the antegrade alignment of the graft, the short length of the graft, and the elimination of any requirement for dissecting or mobilizing the infrarenal aorta. The approach for preparing the field for an aorta to celiac artery graft is simple to accomplish. Preparation for an antegrade bifurcation graft is only slightly more time consuming.

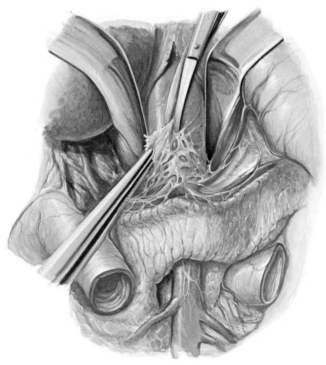 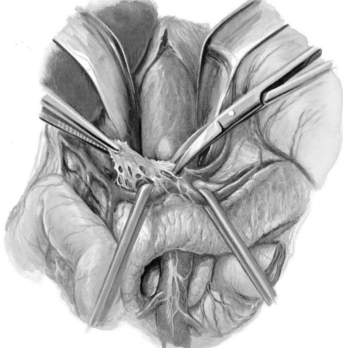

Fig. 7.3. Resection of the supraceliac fibers of the celiac plexus.

Fig. 7.4. Resection of the periceliac fibers. The distal branches of the celiac artery have been mobilized.

212

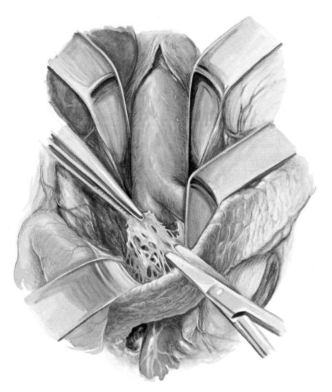

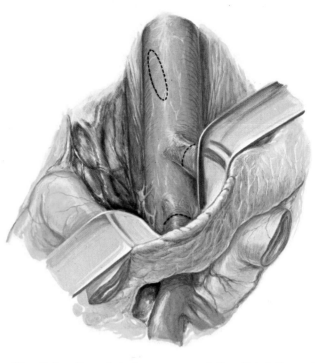

Fig. 7.5. Resection of the celiac ganglion between the celiac artery and the SMA. Note the ease of caudad retraction of the body of the pancreas.

Fig. 7.6. Completed exposure of the distal thoracic aorta and both proximal visceral branches. The proximal aortotomy is placed at an oblique angle on the right anterolateral aspect of the aorta to favor the alignment of the graft limbs. The proximal anastomosis is made between two aortic clamps, both placed proximal to the celiac arteries. Restricting aortic clamping to this segment avoids the potential complications from intimal disruption that can result from aortic clamping at a more distal level.

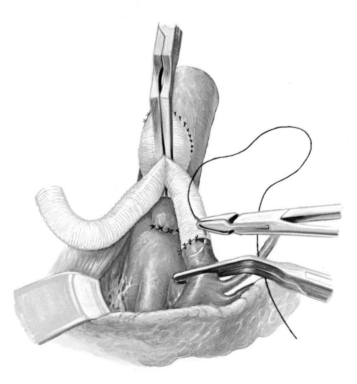

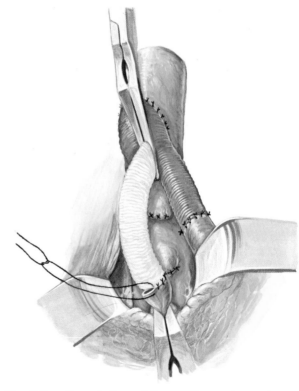

Fig. 7.7. Aortic anastomosis complete and celiac anastomosis in progress. Aortic flow has been restored. In these and subsequent drawings the nonfunctioning portions of the graft are pictured in white for purposes of clarity even though they have been preclotted.

Fig. 7.8. Completion of the SMA anastomosis.

213

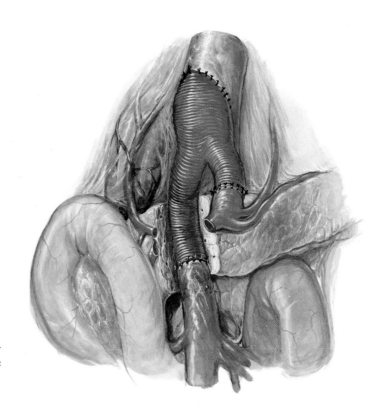

Fig. 7.9. Final alignment of the graft with the artist's cutaway of a section of pancreas to show the retropancreatic course of the SMA limb.

Visceral Artery Endarterectomy

On theoretic grounds, endarterectomy is particularly suited for revascularization of visceral arteries that are stenosed or occluded by atherosclerosis. The primary visceral artery portion of the lesion is confined to the orifice, and the end point is an abrupt one. In this respect, the lesions are comparable to those in the internal carotid and vertebral arteries. When occlusion is complete, the distal propagation of thrombus extends for only a short distance and the arterial tree beyond that point is normal. In the past, the major deterrent to this operation was the difficulty in surgical approach. Because of this, early operations were performed through arteriotomies in the diseased artery. These were largely unsuccessful because of the problem in removing the thick layer of diseased aortic intima surrounding the visceral artery orifice. The frequency of early thrombosis suggested that the ragged ledge of aortic intima produced undesirable turbulence.

In order to overcome this problem, we turned to transaortic endarterectomy in an attempt to utilize the method shown to be successful for atherosclerotic renal artery lesions. Although the results from the limited number of operations we performed through an abdominal approach were durable, the difficulties in obtaining safe access were often formidable.

Thoracoabdominal Retroperitoneal Approach

Modification of the approach by the use of the thoracoabdominal retroperitoneal route has overcome most of the previous problems and is the method with which we currently have the longest experience. The approach lends itself to the safe performance of several possible reconstructive requirements, e.g., opening the orifices of the celiac and SMA, removing obstructing lesions in the renal arteries, and dealing with associated obstructive or aneurysmal disease in the infrarenal aorta.

214

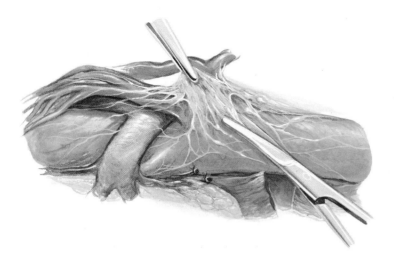

Fig. 7.10. Neural plexus on surface of aorta.

The first stage of the operation requires resection of the dense neural plexus encasing the anterior half of the aorta (**Fig. 7.10**). When only the celiac and SMA are involved, a "trapdoor" aortotomy surrounding the two arterial orifices allows removal of the anterior aortic intima along with the orifice lesions in the visceral branches. If the aortic atheroma is confined to the anterior aorta, the endarterectomy is limited to the under surface of the trapdoor (**Fig. 7.11a–d**). When extensive atheromatous disease involves the full circumference of the aorta, a sleeve of the aortic intima in this segment is removed. Although a projecting ledge of thickened intima will remain at the distal aortic end point, this has never resulted in complications from obstruction or intramural dissection. The reader is referred to Chapter 2 for a description of the technical details of transaortic branch artery endarterectomy.

When the SMA is totally occluded it is possible to remove the atherosclerotic portion of the lesion through aortotomy. The end point of the "tail thrombus" cannot be reached through this approach alone. The

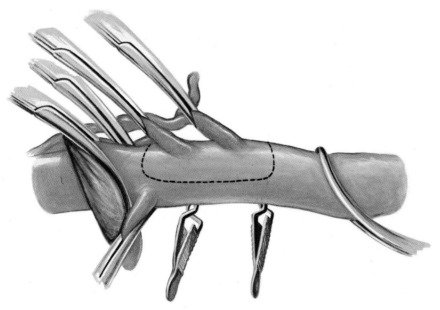

a trapdoor aortotomy

Fig. 7.11,a–d. Transaortic endarterectomy for celiac and superior mesenteric stenosis.

215

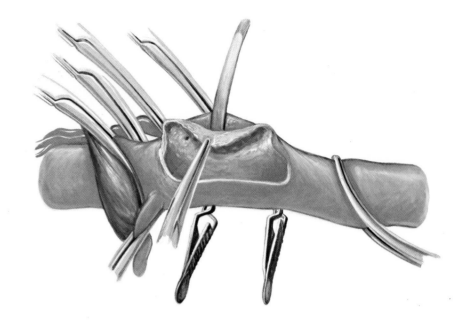

Fig. 7.11 (cont.)

b beginning of endarterectomy

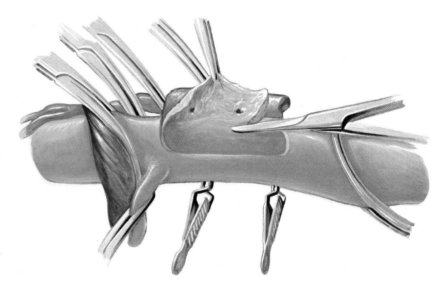

c resection of anterior aortic intima

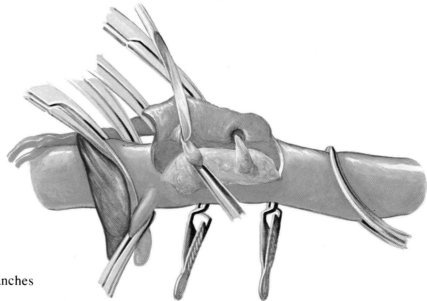

d removal of orifice lesions from branches

216

thrombotic portion of the occlusion extends to the level of the first major branch, 5–8 cm from the origin. The most effective means of management is to remove the orifice lesion during the transaortic portion of the operation, and then to close the aortotomy and restore renal and distal blood flow. The SMA is then clamped across its endarterectomized origin. A longitudinal aortotomy is made to a point just beyond the end of the occlusion. The thrombus is removed by endarterectomy (**Fig. 7.12a**) and the arteriotomy closed with a supplemental vein patch (**Fig. 7.12b**).

Of our patients, 20% have required extension of the operation to deal with renal or infrarenal aortic disease. When renal artery stenosis is present, the longitudinal portion of the aortotomy is merely extended to an infrarenal level (**Fig. 7.13a**) to allow for the performance of renal endarterectomy (**Fig. 7.13b**). Distal aortic occlusive disease is managed by either endarterectomy or bypass graft. If a graft is to be used, it is preferable to transect the aorta slightly distal to the end of the closed aortotomy and to extract the intima from the intact distal aortic stump in preparation for the aorta–graft anastomosis.

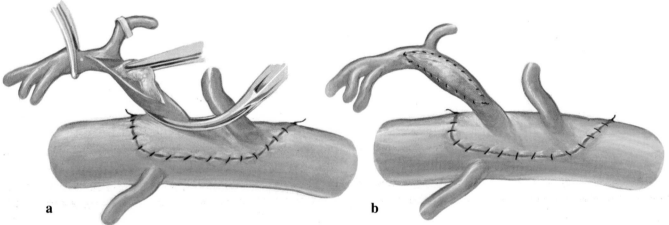

Fig. 7.12,a, b.   Associated total occlusion of superior mesenteric artery. **a** after completion of transaortic endarterectomy (Fig. 7.11), SMA endarterectomy completed through separate incision; **b** vein patch closure.

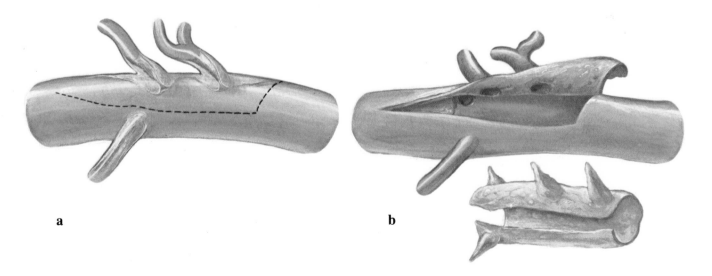

Fig. 7.13,a, b.   Combined visceral and renal endarterectomy. **a** aortotomy; **b** endarterectomy completed and specimen removed.

The transaortic endarterectomy operation for atherosclerotic visceral artery disease by the thoracoabdominal route, which has been used extensively over the past 10 years, has been the most satisfactory procedure of any that we have applied to a large number of patients. Late reocclusion (at 3 months and 3½ years) has occurred in only 2 of the 35 patients who have undergone this procedure. The grafting operation to the celiac artery and the SMA appears to have the potential for the same degree of success. Its use does not preclude combining it with a conventional reconstruction operation in the renal or distal vessels, which is necessary in 20% of the patients. It is estimated that another 10 years of experience will be necessary before the merits of the two operative technics can be compared.

Transperitoneal Approach

Thrombosis superimposed upon a chronic atherosclerotic lesion in either the SMA or the celiac artery may occur as an acute event resulting in intestinal infarction. Acute hypovolemia from any cause may also precipitate intestinal infarction when chronic visceral artery stenosis is present. In both situations, advanced atherosclerotic lesions are often found in both arteries.

This is one circumstance in which endarterectomy from a purely abdominal approach may be the most expeditious technique. The nature of the vascular lesions is often discovered after a laparotomy has been performed for the surgical management of bowel necrosis. Except for cases of frank gangrene of the entire small intestine, revascularization may be effective in decreasing the length of intestine that must be resected. The septic field precludes the use of fabric grafts. Autogenous grafts (e.g., the saphenous vein) or endarterectomy are the only applicable techniques.

Although more difficult than through the thoracoabdominal approach described above, endarterectomy of the celiac artery can be accomplished through the anterior approach used for aortoceliac grafts. The lesion may be removed through a local trapdoor aortotomy partially surrounding the celiac orifice. In one patient, a complete disk of the aorta that included the celiac artery was excised to simplify the endarterectomy and then returned to the aorta after the intima had been removed from its undersurface and the orifice of the celiac artery.

Our limited experience with the use of this operation when necrosis of a portion of the small intestine has already developed suggests that when both arteries are occluded, celiac revascularization alone will usually be adequate to restore sufficient blood flow to the intestine bordering the infarcted segment. Should this fail to occur or should only the SMA be diseased, a similar operation, with a vein patch angioplasty if necessary, can be performed at the SMA orifice.

The preceding comments can be placed in clinical perspective when one considers the problems of the patient with known visceral artery lesions who requires an emergent operation for suspected impending or frank infarction of the intestine. (This situation may develop following an extensive arteriography procedure in a patient under study for chronic visceral ischemia.) A transperitoneal approach is needed in the event that portions of the intestine may require resection. If infarction is not present and combined lesions in the celiac and SMA are present, one of the two grafting operations may be performed depending on the patient's general condition. If frank or near infarction is present and an intestinal operation seems required, a preliminary revascularization of the celiac or SMA may be performed by transaortic endarterectomy through the abdomen. (Synthetic grafts in this situation are contraindicated.) This may substantially lessen the length of intestine requiring resection.

With either operative method there may remain segments of intestine with marginal blood supply. In this circumstance, a "second look" operation 24 hours later is generally advisable.

The following photographs and aortograms (**Figs. 7.14–7.26**) illustrate the implications of the natural history and variations in the clinical presentation and the arterial lesions seen during surgical management of chronic visceral ischemia.

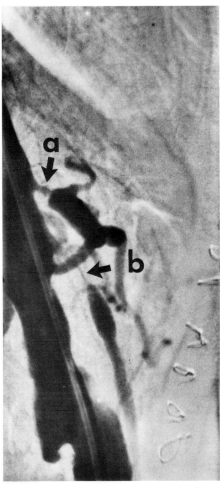

a

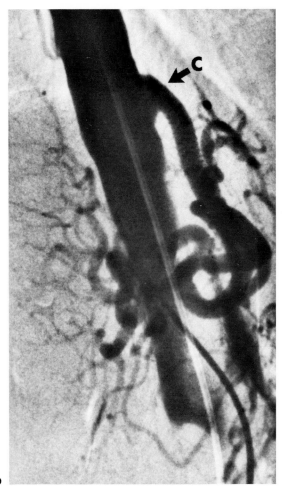

b

Fig. 7.14,a, b. Lateral aortograms (a preoperative; b postoperative) in a patient with a Dacron bypass graft to the celiac artery. This patient had undergone an aortofemoral bypass graft operation 7 years before. The proximal end of the old aortic graft is visible at the bottom of the preoperative film. Note severe stenosis at the orifice of the celiac artery (a) and near occlusion of the SMA, the lumen of which has been reduced to the size of a string in its proximal 3 cm (b).

The patient developed acute abdominal pain a few hours after the aortogram, and an emergency operation was performed. The small intestine was dusky but not infarcted. Operation was limited to celiac re-vascularization. A 6-mm flanged graft was anastomosed end-to-side to the supraceliac aorta and end-to-end to the transected celiac artery. In the postoperative film, note the bell-shaped orifice of the graft (c), which has been cut from a 10 × 5-mm knitted Dacron bifurcation graft, and the rapid collateral filling of the terminal branches of the still-stenosed SMA. The still-patent aorta graft had not filled at the time this exposure was made. Normal color returned to the intestine immediately following restoration of normal blood flow in the celiac artery. The patient has remained symptom-free for 2 years.

219

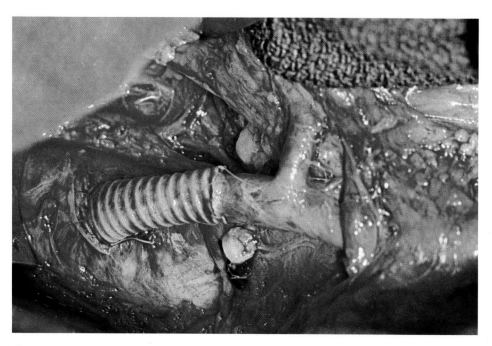

Fig. 7.15. Operative photograph of an aortoceliac 6-mm bypass graft in a poor-risk acutely ill patient with chronic visceral ischemia and atherosclerotic stenosis of the SMA and the celiac artery (patient's head to the left). The ligated stump of the celiac artery and the lesion within it are visible in the center of the photograph.

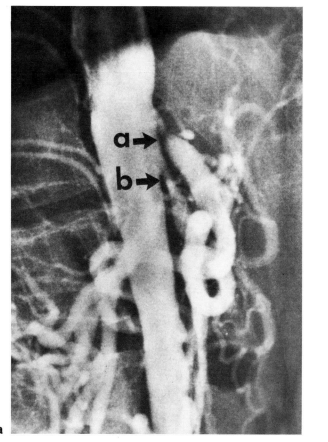

a

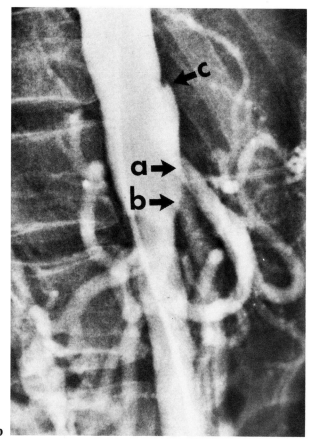

b

Fig. 7.16,a, b. Aortograms (**a** preoperative; **b** postoperative) in the lateral projection showing atherosclerotic stenosis of the celiac (*a*) and superior mesenteric (*b*) arteries. A sleeve of aortic intima, including the orifice lesions in the stenosed arteries, has been removed. In the postoperative aortagram, note the upper level of aortic endarterectomy at *c*.

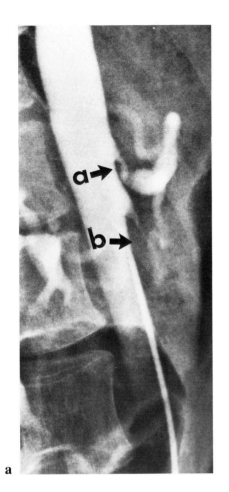

a

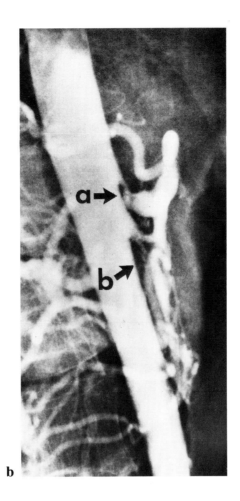

b

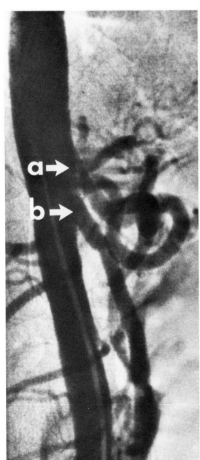

c

Fig. 7.17,a–c. Serial aortograms (**a**, **b** preoperative; **c** postoperative) in the lateral projection in a patient with atherosclerotic stenosis of the celiac (*a*) and superior mesenteric (*b*) arteries. Results of transaortic endarterectomy are shown in postoperative aortogram.

221

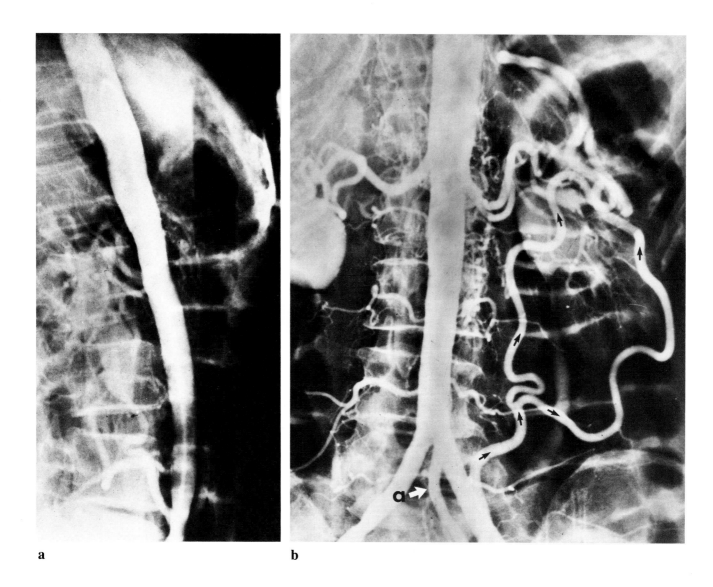

a   b

Fig. 7.18,a–d. Midstream aortograms (**a, b** preoperative; **c, d** postoperative) in a patient with atherosclerotic occlusion of the SMA and celiac arteries. In the lateral projection (**a**) the only patent anterior branch of the aorta is the IMA. In the P-A projection (**b**) the left colic branches of the IMA have become a major source of collateral blood supply to the proximal viscera and are seen extending toward their connections with the SMA (*serial arrows*). The proximal IMA has become abnormally enlarged (*a*).

At operation, a sleeve endarterectomy of the aorta to include the orifice lesions in the celiac and SMA was performed. Because of difficulty with the end point in the celiac artery, a Dacron graft beginning in the distal thoracic aorta was used to replace it. The postoperative aortograms from the lateral (**c**) and AP (**d**) projections demonstrate normal forward flow with both the celiac and superior mesenteric arteries. The origin of the celiac graft is demonstrated (*b*). The technique shown in Figs. 7.12a and b and 7.22a was used to reopen the occluded SMA.

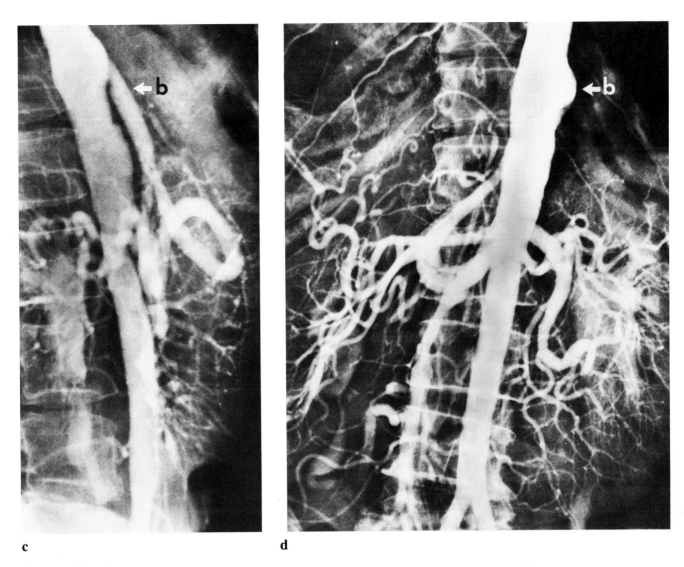

c

d

Fig. 7.18 (cont.)

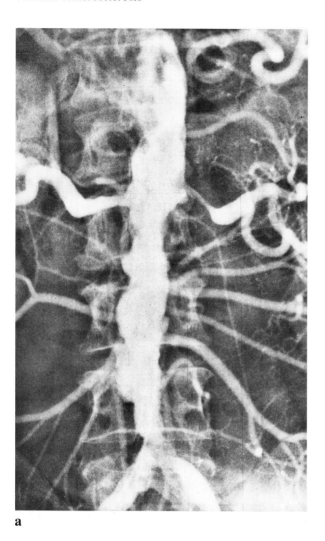

a

Fig. 7.19, a–c. Aortogram (**a**) in a patient with hypertension and chronic visceral ischemia showing diffuse degenerative atherosclerosis in the infrarenal aorta, bilateral renal artery stenosis, and intraluminal filling defects in the suprarenal aorta. Not shown is stenosis of the celiac artery and SMA. Operation was performed through a thoracoabdominal approach. Transaortic endarterectomy removed the aortic intima from the celiac artery superiorly to beyond the renal arteries inferiorly and included orifice lesions in the two visceral and two renal arteries. The infrarenal aorta was replaced by a Dacron graft. **b** The closed aortotomy and the graft in place. **c** Photograph of resected specimen showing massive accumulation of mural thrombus in the suprarenal aorta, the orifice lesion in the SMA (middle, left), and the lesions removed from the renal arteries (bottom, right and left).

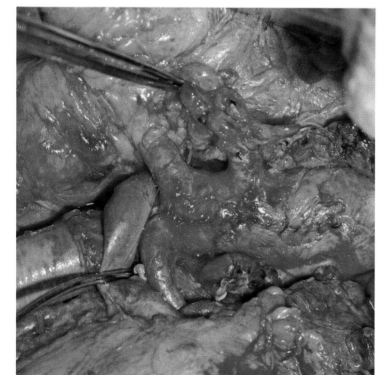

b

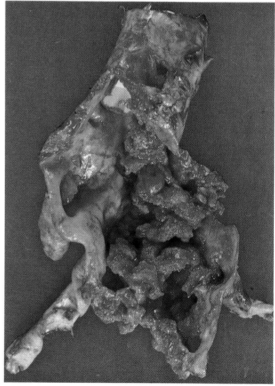

c

224

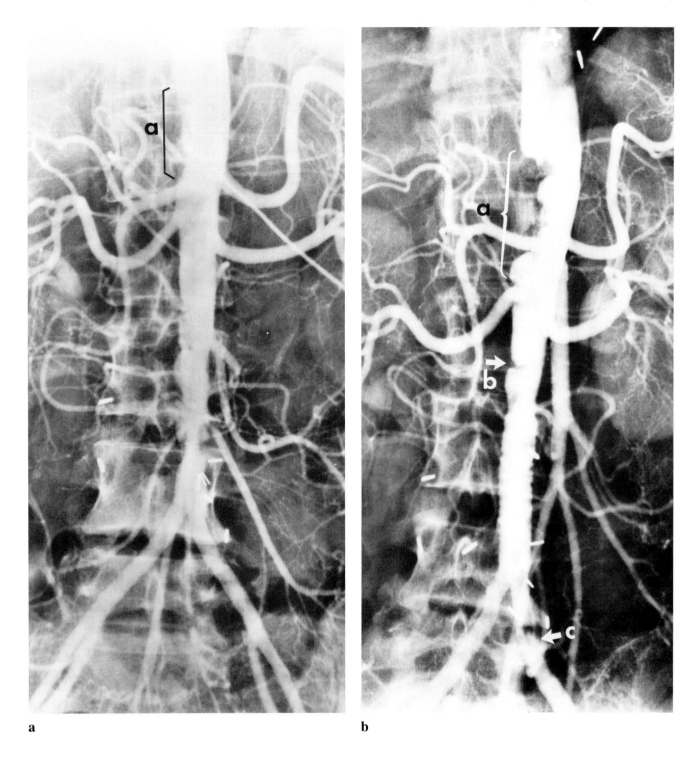

a   b

Fig. 7.20,a–c. Aortogram (**a**) in a 42-year-old woman with disabling claudication caused by infrarenal atherosclerosic stenosis of the aorta. Note the small irregular filling defect in the right side of the aorta proximal to the renal arteries (*a*). A tubular graft was used to replace the distal two-thirds of the infrarenal aorta. Aortogram taken five years later (**b**) after symptoms of chronic visceral ischemia have appeared and claudication has recurred in the left leg. Note the now-large filling defect in the suprarenal aorta (*a*). Atherosclerosis has developed in the infrarenal aortic stump (*b*) and in the left common iliac artery (*c*). The latter two lesions could have been prevented if the surgeon had taken into account the pattern of progression of atherosclerosis in the infrarenal aorta and the iliac arteries and had performed a more extensive operation. (Part **c** appears on the next page.)

225

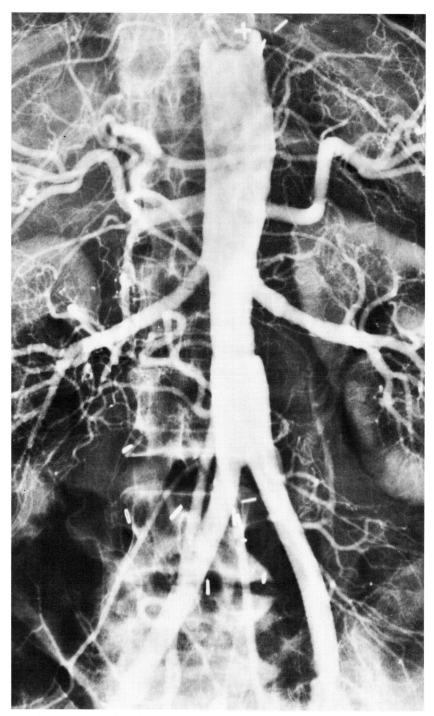

Fig. 7.20c. Aortogram following a second operation. Endarterectomy of the aorta through a thoracoabdominal (retroperitoneal) approach from the level of the diaphragm to a level 4 cm distal to the renal arteries which removed orifice lesions in the celiac artery and SMA has been performed. A bifurcation graft (14 × 7) was used to replace the previous graft and the common iliac arteries.

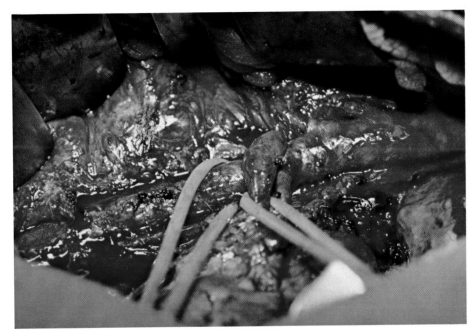

a

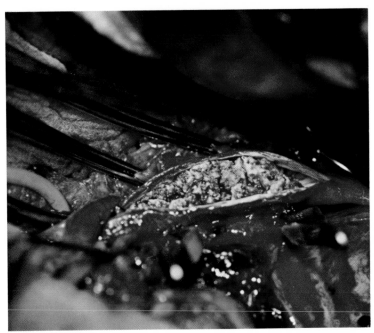

b

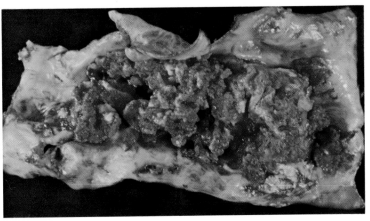

c

Fig. 7.21. a Exposure for the operation described in Fig. 7.20c. The patient's head is to the right. **b** Interior of the suprarenal aorta. The clamps at the top are on the celiac and SMA. **c** Endarterectomy specimen showing the cauliflower atheromatous mass in the aorta and the orifice lesion in the SMA (at the top). [From Stoney RJ, Ehrenfeld WK, Wylie EJ: Revascularization methods in chronic visceral ischemia caused by atherosclerosis. Ann Surg, 186 (4):468–476, October 1977.]

227

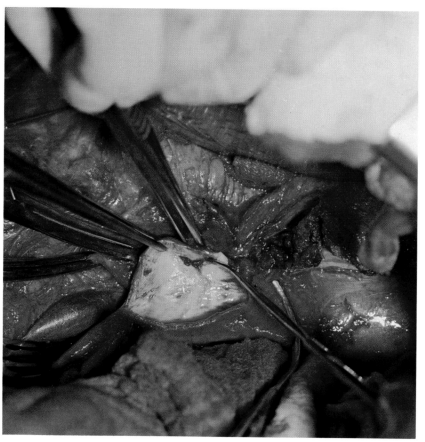

a

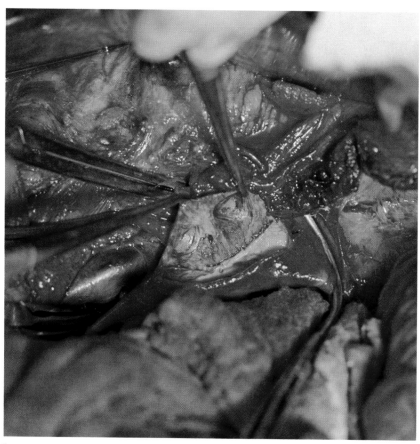

Fig. 7.22a, b. Operative photographs during transaortic endarterectomy for atherosclerotic stenosis of the SMA and celiac arteries. **a** A trapdoor incision that raises a flap containing the origins of the stenotic arteries has been made in the suprarenal aorta. The celiac clamp has been released. A drop of blood is visible coming from a 1-mm opening in the aorta. The SMA orifice is barely visible. Illustrated are the type of lesions in which the buttery aortic intima seems almost to "overflow" the branching arteries. The left renal vein can be seen crossing the aorta at the left side of the photograph. **b** The endarterectomy has been confined to the anterior surface of the aorta adjacent to the visceral branches. The orifices of the SMA and celiac arteries have been restored to a normal size.

b

228

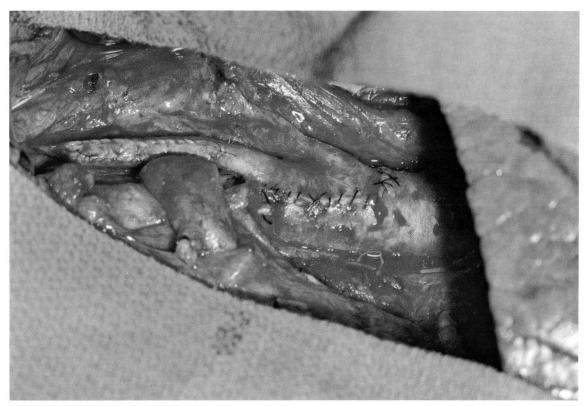

a

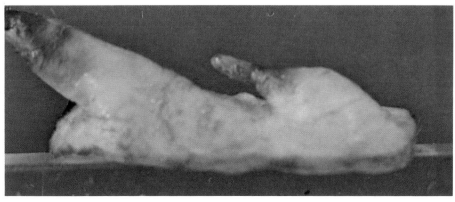

b

Fig. 7.23,a–c. Photographs of the operative field (**a**) and the endarterectomy specimen (**b**, **c**) following transaortic endarterectomy for celiac stenosis and SMA occlusion (patient's head is to the right). The primary atherosclerotic lesion in the SMA was confined to its orifice but thrombosis had extended distally to the level of origin of the first major branch that arises from the side of the artery opposite to the side shown and is not in view. The thrombus was removed through a longitudinal SMA arteriotomy, which was closed with a supplementary vein patch. This portion of the operation was performed after the aortotomy had been closed and normal flow in the aorta restored. A thoracoretroperitoneal abdominal incision was used. The edge of the left lower lobe of the lung can be seen to the right.

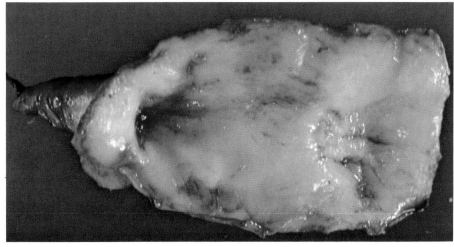

c

229

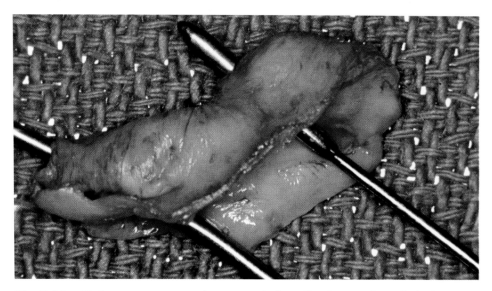

Fig. 7.24. Endarterectomy specimen consisting of a sleeve of aortic intima with probes in the orifices of the celiac artery and the SMA. Note the thick layer of the peculiar succulent intima that is frequently found in the aorta in patients with stenosis or occlusion of the visceral arteries.

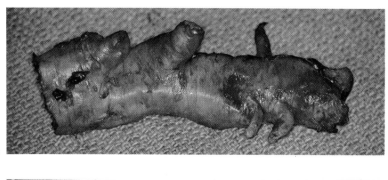

a

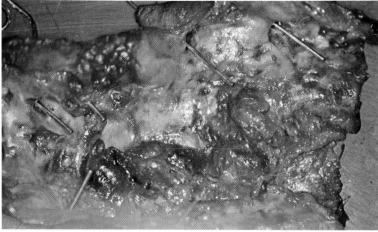

b

Fig. 7.25,a, b. Endarterectomy specimen in a patient with chronic visceral ischemia and renovascular hypertension. Stenosis of three renal arteries as well as the two major visceral arteries was demonstrated on the preoperative aortogram. The exterior surface of the specimen, which has been closed with sutures, is shown in **a**. Note the protruding nubbins of thickened intima that have been removed from the orifices of the SMA and celiac arteries (top) and the three renal arteries (left). The opened specimen (**b**) shows the same succulent intima illustrated in Fig. 7.17. But in this spotty endothelial ulceration has become the focus for attachment of scattered mural thrombus. This type of aortic intimal disease, which is also present in the infrarenal aorta, makes it difficult to use the abdominal aorta as the origin for bypass grafts that are of appropriate size for distal anastomosis.

230

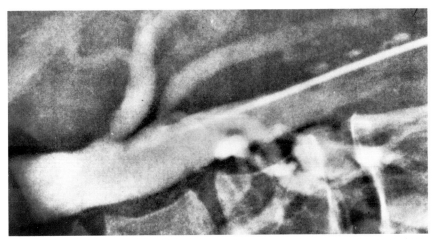

a

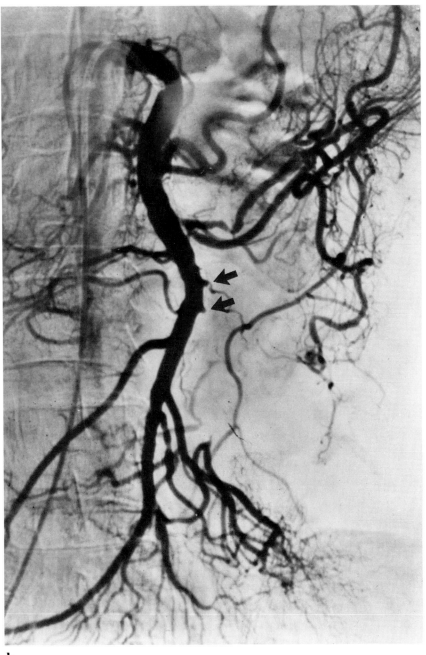

Fig. 7.26a–d. (a) Midstream aortogram (lateral projection) and (b) selective SMA arteriogram in a 47-year-old woman with a 2-month history of abdominal pain characteristic of chronic visceral ischemia and a loud upper abdominal bruit. The aortogram shows stenotic lesions at the orifices of the celiac artery and the SMA. Also shown are flakes of calcium in the anterior wall of the intra-renal aorta. The film of the SMA shows occlusion of at least two of the distal branches (*arrows*). Twelve hours after the arteriogram, the patient developed progressively severe abdominal pain and signs of increasing peritoneal irritation. Emergency laparotomy disclosed generalized ischemia of the small intestine maximum in the segment of jejunum peripheral to two yellow, calcified and pulseless mesenteric arteries. Orifice lesions and distal thrills were palpable in both the celiac artery and the SMA. In the absence of bacterial contamination a revascularization operation using a fabric graft was feasible. The distal SMA branch artery lesions suggested the need for reopening the proximal SMA as well as the celiac artery. A bifurcation graft to both arteries was implanted by the method shown in Figs. 7.3 to 7.9. (Parts **c** and **d** appear on the next page.)

b

231

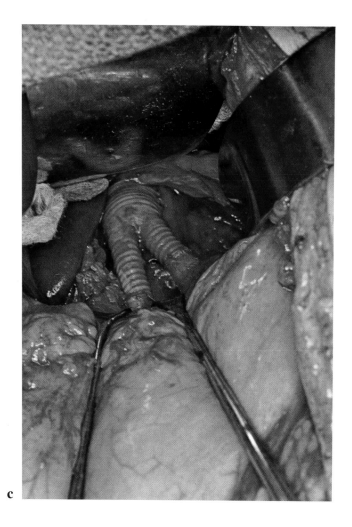

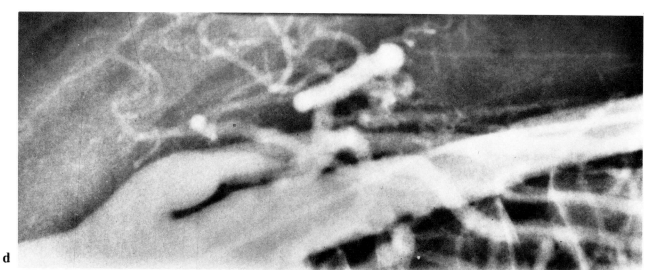

Fig. 7.26. **c** Operative photograph showing the 12 × 6-mm knitted Dacron bifurcation graft in place. Caudad retraction of the stomach and pancreas has made it possible to establish both distal anastomoses from a single approach through the lesser sac. **d** Postoperative lateral aortogram. Satisfactory revascularization, confirmed by a second look operation after 24 hours, had been accomplished.

Renovascular Atherosclerosis

8

The pathologic pattern of atherosclerosis in patients with renal artery atherosclerosis is similar in many respects to that found in patients with visceral artery atherosclerotic lesions. The arterial lesion is generally confined to the proximal third of the artery and tends to come to an abrupt end, sparing the distal intima. Although the stenosis in one renal artery may predominate, lesser degrees of orifice lesions will usually be present in the opposite renal artery and any accessory renal arteries that may be present. The progression of these associated lesions tends in time to nullify the results of a successful operation directed solely to the blood supply of the kidney originally responsible for the hypertension. Thus, in the patient with atherosclerosis, the identification of the kidney responsible for the hypertension becomes more academic than practical if one is selecting an operation that is most likely to produce sustained relief of hypertension.

The aortic intima both proximal and distal to the renal arteries is almost invariably thickened by atherosclerosis. When viewed from inside the aorta, the aortic intimal disease seems, as with visceral artery lesions, almost to overflow the renal orifices. In the most favorable situation, the aortic intima has a smooth surface and has not thickened to the degree of restricting blood flow through any portion of the infrarenal aorta.

Approximately 20% of patients will have more advanced aortic disease, which influences the extent and the type of operation. This may take the form of obstructive aortoiliac disease. In other patients there may be extensive degenerative disease involving deeper layers of the aortic wall. In this latter group the contour of the infrarenal aorta may vary from irregular zones of minimal aortic widening to frank aneurysm. In most patients with this type of degenerative aortic disease, the aortic intima both distal to and proximal to the renal orifices often becomes a granular necrotic layer, and aortic clamps applied in this area may dislodge masses of this material that can embolize into the renal vascular bed unless appropriate precautions are taken. A preoperative aortogram which shows any degree of widening of the aortic lumen should lead one to anticipate that these changes are present.

The indications for revascularization in a patient with an arteriographically demonstrated renal artery atherosclerotic lesion have undergone critical reevaluation. From the distillation of the numerous investigative studies three basic, and still not totally resolvable, questions become applicable to each clinical situation. First, does the presence of a lesion indicate that the hypertension is the result of the lesion? Of all the various studies, the arteriographic demonstration of a hemodynamically significant lesion continues, in our experience, to be as reliable as any of the other studies in predicting that the hypertension is of renovascular origin. When the midstream aortic injection demonstrates collateral vessels, such as those surrounding the ureter, supplying the kidney, one can be certain that the renal artery lesion is hemodynamically significant. Although the predictability of arteriography is less than certain, efforts to find studies with greater accuracy have been less fruitful.

Second, will removal of the lesion have a substantial chance of lessening the hypertension? In our experience, the probability of a successful outcome is greater than 70% if operation is limited to patients in a young age group (<60 years) and without extensive atherosclerosis at other sites.

Third, and most important, will lowering of blood pressure by operation result in prolongation of life? Since the hypertension itself is usually asymptomatic in most of these patients, potential extension of longevity by removal of the lesion becomes the only real indication for operation. Elderly patients with renovascular hypertension caused by atherosclerosis have a limited longevity because of atherosclerosis at other sites and the variety of other afflictions to which they are susceptible. Except for those patients with early or impending uremia as a result of severe bilateral renal artery lesions, the possibility of substantial prolongation of the life of an elderly patient by a technically successful renal artery reconstructive operation is slim. On the other hand, younger patients with severe hypertension, even though medically controllable, become surgical candidates because of the undesirable side-effects and inconstancy of blood pressure control even with the more vigorous medical regimens. In this group, the sustained reduction of blood pressure levels to normal or near normal by a successful operation would clearly appear to extend longevity.

Bypass Grafting

Perhaps the most commonly used operation is the placement of a bypass fabric prosthesis from the side of the aorta distal to the renal arteries that is extended in a retrograde direction to the side of the renal artery distal to the lesion. This technique is not applicable for those patients who have the degenerative form of aortic disease described above unless it is combined with resection of the infrarenal aorta, in which case a side arm from the aortic prosthesis may be used to revascularize the kidney.

There are several major drawbacks to the uniform use of a simple aortorenal graft. The thickened aortic wall poses mechanical problems in creating a satisfactory proximal anastomosis without using an oversized graft (i.e., one larger than the renal artery). Distally, both the disparity in graft–artery size and the redirection of flow direction by an end-to-side anastomosis are conducive to graft thrombosis. Proximally, the inevitable advance of the aortic atherosclerosis becomes a constant threat to eventual closure of the proximal anastomosis.

These problems can be partially overcome by the use of a smaller graft (5–6 cm) cut from a bifurcation graft to provide a flange for the proximal anastomosis and the use of an end-to-end anastomosis at the distal end. Regardless of its refinements, this technique is applicable only for those patients with large, paired renal arteries with only minimal disease in the infrarenal aorta, and it is not a technique applicable to patients with associated lesions in smaller accessory arteries.

Endarterectomy

The alternative to bypass grafting in the usual pathologic situation, and the one we prefer, is endarterectomy. Early in our experience, we attempted endarterectomy through transverse arteriotomies in the renal arteries near their origins. Although this approach was often successful, we frequently encountered difficulties in removing the thickened aortic intima surrounding the renal orifice. Endarterectomy through a longitudinal renal arteriotomy extending onto the aorta with patch graft closure has been an unsuitable compromise because of the difficulty in providing a vessel with an even contour. We subsequently turned to the currently employed operation of endarterectomy from within the opened aorta. This technique removes all of the aortic intima above and below the renal orifices.

Although technically more demanding than the bypass graft techniques, the improved immediate and long-term results have shown endarterectomy from within to be the superior technique in our hands. The aorta is approached through the standard longitudinal abdominal incision. A flank incision provides access to only one renal artery and is not adequate for an operation that usually should include both renal arteries and often the management of infrarenal aortic lesions in addition.

The tedious and time-consuming portion of the operation is the mobilization of the aorta and the renal arteries. The superior mesenteric artery often arises close to the level of the renal arteries. Since a successful operation required exposure of the interior of the aorta above (as well as below) the renal arteries, the aortotomy must be extended proximally to the level of, or just cephalad to, the SMA. This can only be accomplished if the aorta has been mobilized to the level of the celiac artery and the dense mass of neural tissue on the anterior surface of the aorta between the celiac and superior mesenteric arteries has been dissected free of the aorta. It is then possible to crossclamp the aorta proximal to the SMA with ease and safety.

Mobilization of the suprarenal aorta is simplified if fibers of the origin of diaphragmatic crura are cut. These fibers can be identified by palpation of the tight musculotendinous ridges closely adherent to the posterior halves of the side of the aorta. Once these fibers have been cut (**Fig. 8.1a**), exposure of the posterolateral aspects of the proximal aorta is accomplished by blunt finger dissection (**Fig. 8.1b and c**).

The small adrenal arteries, which arise from each side of the aorta at the level of the SMA, should be divided and tied before advancing the finger along the side of, and posterior to, the aorta. This portion of the operation is complete when openings have been developed for application of an occluding clamp across the aorta between the SMA and celiac arteries.

The two pairs of lumbar arteries are occluded by inserting the jaws of a long, straight aorta clamp from below and into the planes on each side of the aorta created by the finger dissection. Closure of the jaws of the clamp compresses all of the tissue posterior to the aorta in one maneuver and avoids the hazard of attempting to control each lumbar artery individually (**Fig. 8.2**).

235

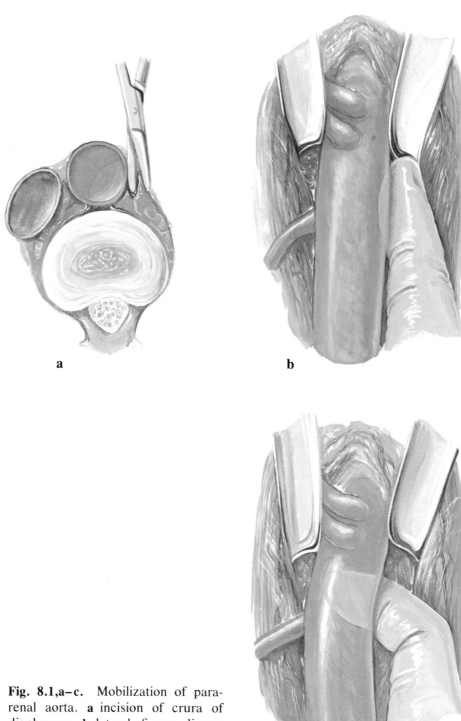

Fig. 8.1,a–c. Mobilization of para-renal aorta. **a** incision of crura of diaphragm; **b** lateral finger dissection; **c** retroaortic dissection.

Clamps are then applied individually to the SMA, the renal arteries distal to the atheroma, and to the aorta proximal and distal to the site of the proposed aortotomy (**Fig. 8.3**). The distal aorta is carefully palpated and is clamped at a level of minimal thickness of the aortic wall, usually just cephalad to the IMA. More recently, we have been impressed with the relative ease of an alternate technique, the application of the proximal aortic clamp cephalad to the celiac artery. This portion of the aorta is readily accessible by an approach through the gastrohepatic ligament, followed by splitting of the posterior fibers of the diaphragm. Clamping of the aorta at this level provides an almost bloodless field when the aortotomy is made.

An 8–10 cm aortotomy is then made on the anterior surface of the aorta and extended proximally in a line midway between the renal arteries. The cephalad end of the aortotomy is curved to the left of the superior mesenteric artery and terminated at a point just proximal to it.

The basic maneuver for endarterectomy in this operation is the removal of a sleeve of the entire aortic intima, taking with it the orifice lesions in all of the renal arteries. This is accomplished by first transecting the aortic intima distally at a point of the least intimal thickening. Although this leaves a ledge of thickened intima distally, we have encountered no complications of distal dissection and tack-down sutures are not necessary. The aortic endarterectomy is then extended proximally. The entire aortic intima should first be dissected free before approaching the portion adjacent to the renal orifices. The proximal end of the aortic intimal sleeve is transected with scissors immediately distal to the SMA orifice (**Fig. 8.4**). Extension of the endarterectomy to a higher level creates the possibility of postoperative dissection into the wall of the SMA.

The renal lesions are then approached individually. With forceps on the freed aortic intima, the dissecting instrument gently pushes away the media of the renal artery in a maneuver that eventually creates an eversion

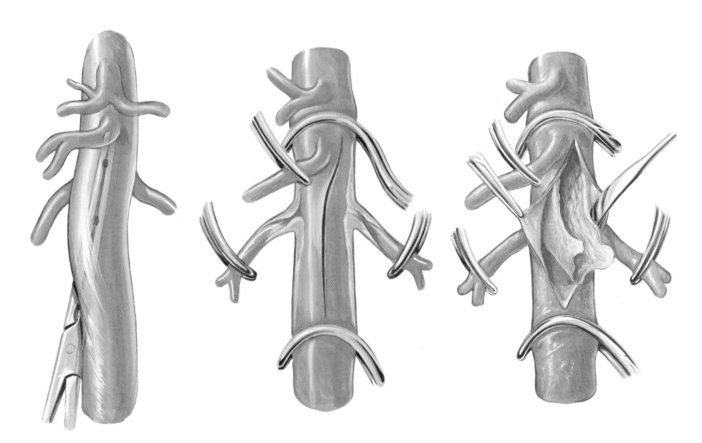

Fig. 8.2. Occlusion of lumbar arteries.

Fig. 8.3. Aortotomy for transaortic renal endarterectomy.

Fig. 8.4. Preliminary aortic endarterectomy.

237

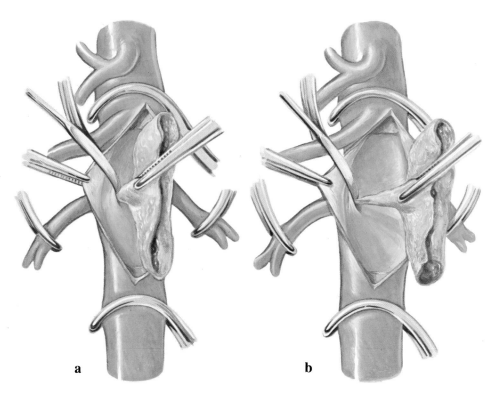

a   b

Fig. 8.5,a, b.   Removal of renal lesions. **a** dissection in endarterectomy plane in right renal artery after aortic portion has been completed; **b** end point of renal endarterectomy.

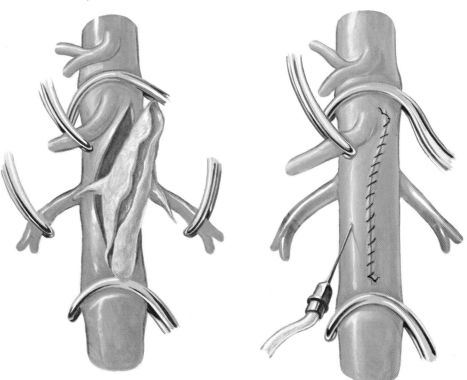

Fig. 8.6.   Endarterectomy completed.

Fig. 8.7.   Procedure for operative arteriogram.

238

endarterectomy as the renal artery prolapses into the aortic lumen (**Fig. 8.5a and b**). The first assistant can be helpful at this time by using a hand in the lateral gutter to dislocate the kidney to a more medial position. As the end point of the renal lesion is approached, the specimen breaks free, leaving an end point similar to that observed with carotid endarterectomy (**Fig. 8.6**). (See Chapter 2, p. 30, for variations in technique.)

After extraction of residual intimal fragments and the customary flushing and backbleeding by momentary and alternate release of the proximal and distal aortic clamps, the aortotomy is closed with a continuous suture of 4–0 silk. The renal ischemia time will rarely exceed 15–20 min, a time period that permits restoration of a normal lumen to all of the renal arteries without exceeding the limit of safe renal ischemia.

The final step in the operation is assessment of the adequacy of the renal endarterectomy end points, determined by finger compression of the renal arteries supplemented by an operative arteriogram. Operative arteriograms of adequate clarity require replacement of the proximal and distal aortic clamps and injection of contrast solution into the segment of aorta between the clamps (**Fig. 8.7**). If a suspicious lesion is palpated or observed on x-ray, it is removed by endarterectomy through a transverse renal arteriotomy placed just distal to the lesion (**Fig. 8.8a**). The occluding clamp is applied to the involved renal artery at its origin. The posterior intima is incised and a dissection developed to permit removal of the remaining intima in the proximal renal artery (**Fig. 8.8b and c**).

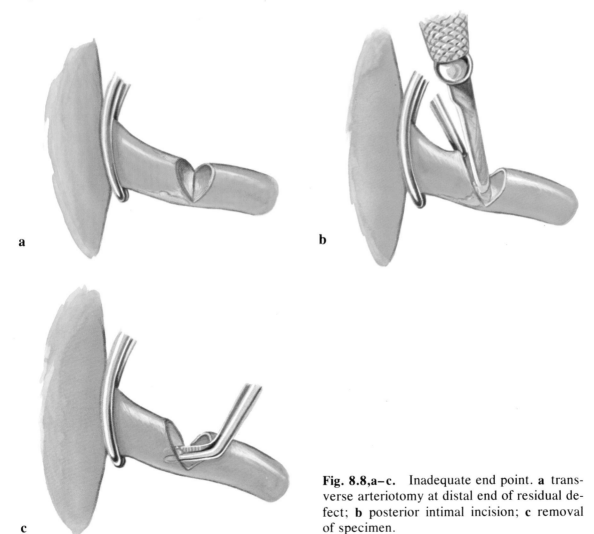

a

b

c

Fig. 8.8,a–c. Inadequate end point. **a** transverse arteriotomy at distal end of residual defect; **b** posterior intimal incision; **c** removal of specimen.

The primary purpose of the operative arteriogram is the delineation of the arterial lumen at the end point of the endarterectomy or the site of a graft anastomosis. Severe and spotty zones of stenosis in the distal arterial branches that are the result of temporary vasoconstriction in an arterial bed particularly vulnerable to this response are often demonstrated. No attempt should be made to extend the operation into these segments, since these irregularities will disappear spontaneously.

Distal aortoiliac disease may require endarterectomy or bypass. Endarterectomy calls for only transferring the suprarenal clamp to an infrarenal position and proceeding as described in Chapter 5. If a bypass graft is to be used, the infrarenal aorta should be transected distal to the lower end of the previous aortotomy. Extraction of the cuff of intima in the interval aortic segment provides an excellent aortic stump for the use of an end-to-end anastomosis to the aortic portion of a bifurcation prosthesis.

Renal endarterectomy is often difficult to perform with safety in patients with the degenerative type of aortic disease described previously. A smooth endarterectomy plane can be reached only by deep penetration of the aortic wall. The end point in the renal artery is less precise. Aortic cross-clamping adjacent to the renal orifices is hazardous. With this type of pathology, graft replacement of the infrarenal aorta is usually advisable. A sidearm prosthetic graft with a flanged end is extended from the aortic prosthesis and anastomosed end-to-end to the transected renal artery. The aorta is clamped proximal to the celiac artery above the level of intimal degeneration to avoid intimal fragmentation in the jaws of the clamp. The infrarenal aorta is transected and the aortic prosthesis (with the side arm in place) is anastomosed to the aortic stump. The aortic clamp is then transferred to an infrarenal position while the distal iliac or femoral anastomoses are completed.

The renal side arm is preferably made with a 5 or 6 mm graft with a flange on the proximal end anastomosed proximally to an elliptical incision on the side of the aortic prosthesis. The use of an end-to-end distal anastomosis minimizes turbulence that an end-to-side anastomosis would produce and lessens the possibility of thrombosis. It is important that the graft be cut to a length that would allow it to assume a natural curve as it aligns itself to the outflow artery. This can be determined by pinching the distal end of the uncut graft while the proximal clamp is released (**Fig. 8.9a**). With the occluding fingers held at the position adjacent to the still-functioning renal artery at the appropriate point for the anastomosis, the most desired alignment of the graft can be estimated before the graft is transected (**Fig. 8.9a and b**). Following completion of the distal anastomosis, the graft should assume a gentle curve to align itself with the outflow artery. The disparity in the diameters of the graft and the temporarily constricted distal artery may occasionally be difficult to overcome. This is one situation where an end-to-end anastomosis of a fabric graft to an artery is more safely performed with interrupted synthetic 6–0 sutures (**Fig. 8.9b**).

Special attention should be paid to the pre- and postoperative fluid and electrolyte management in all renal revascularization operations. Available evidence suggests that preoperative hydration and mannitol-induced diuresis prior to aortic clamping lessens the vulnerability of the kidney to operative ischemia. Postoperatively some degree of tubular malfunction often becomes apparent. This is a temporary phenomenon if the renal ischemia time has been short, but requires correction of the fluid and electrolyte losses that will result.

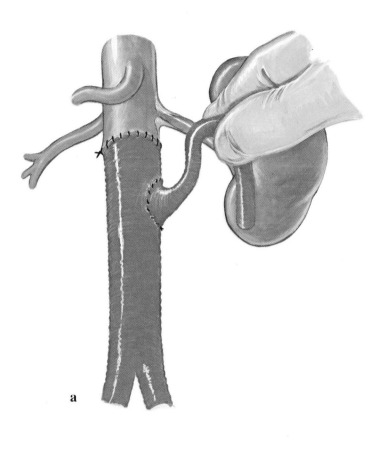

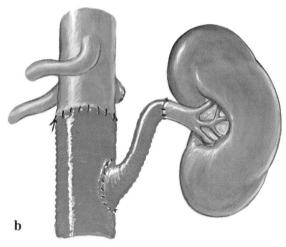

Fig. 8.9,a, b. Aortorenal bypass graft. **a** flanged graft positioned for estimation of optimum length; **b** final alignment with end-to-end distal anastomosis.

The following case histories, photographs and arteriograms **(Figs. 8.10–8.27)** illustrate the implications of the natural history and pathologic variations of renovascular atherosclerotic occlusive disease on various aspects of surgical management.

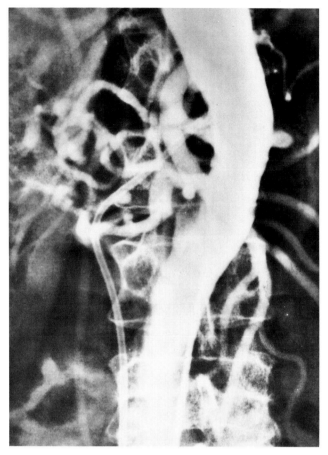

a

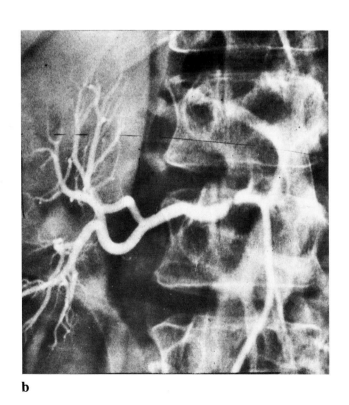

b

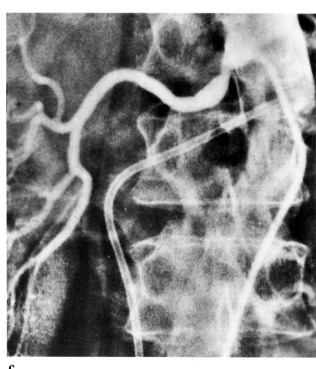

c

Fig. 8.10

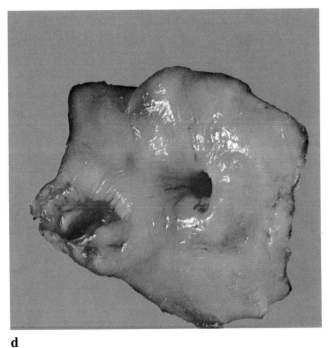

d

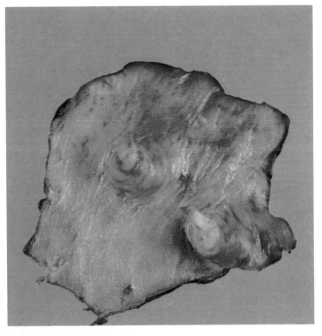

e

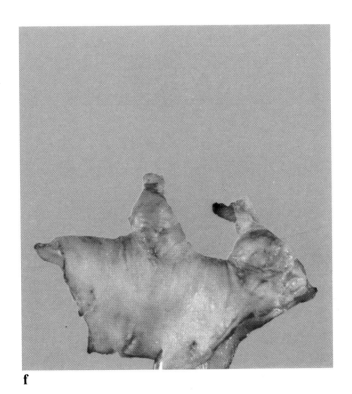

f

Fig. 8.10, a–f. Midstream aortogram (**a**) and selective renal arteriograms (**b, c**) in a 52-year-old woman with uncontrollable hypertension. The aortogram shows thrombosis of the left renal artery but fails to delineate the two right renal arteries because of other overlapping arteries. The selective films show each of these renal arteries, both of which have atherosclerotic lesions at their orifices. The absence of degenerative changes in the aorta and the need for dealing with both arteries simultaneously provides a clear indication for the use of transaortic endarterectomy. Interior (**d**) and exterior (**e, f**) views of specimen removed at operation.

243

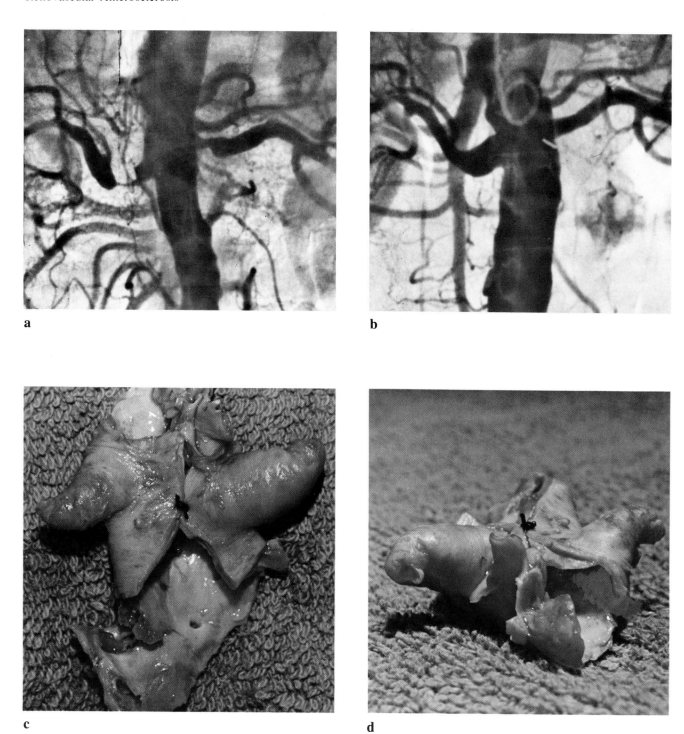

Fig. 8.11,a–d. Aortogram before (**a**) and after (**b**) transaortic renal endarterectomy in a 57-year-old man with hypertension and bilateral renal artery stenosis. **c, d** Two views of an endarterectomy specimen removed at operation. Shown are a sleeve of aortic intima and the lesions removed from the renal arteries.

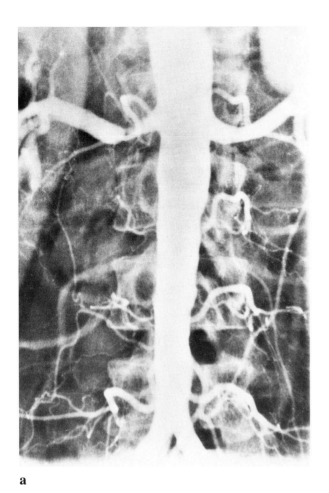

a

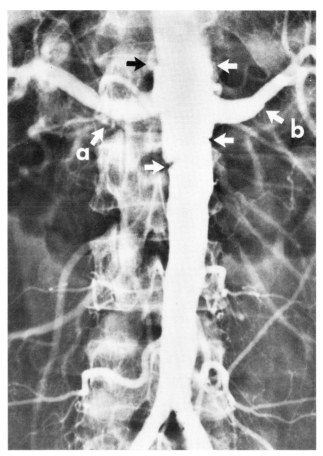

b

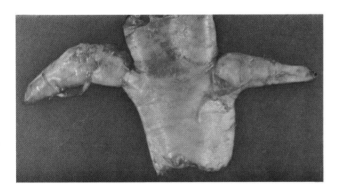

c

d

Fig. 8.12,a–d. Aortograms (**a** preoperative; **b** postoperative) from a patient with hypertension secondary to atherosclerotic stenosis of the right renal artery. The left renal artery contained a ledge of thickened intima posteriorly that was not visible on the aortogram. Transaortic endarterectomy of the pararenal aorta and of the proximal thirds of both renal arteries was performed. The arrows alongside the aorta bracket the aortic portion of the endarterectomy. The end points of the renal portion of the endarterectomy are at *a* and

b. In the surgical specimen (**c, d**) note the generalized succulent thickening of the aortic intima and absence of surface degeneration or fragmentation. This is the type of atherosclerosis that could have been anticipated from inspection of the preoperative aortogram, which displays a smooth, undulating internal contour and narrowing of the diameter of the infrarenal aorta. This type of aortic atherosclerosis simplifies the performance of transaortic endarterectomy for renal and visceral artery stenosis.

245

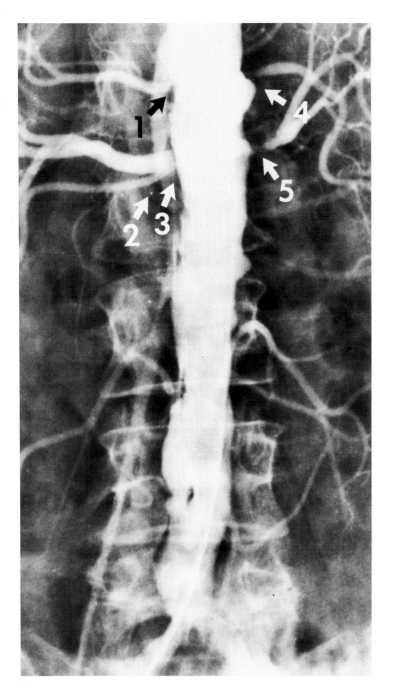

a

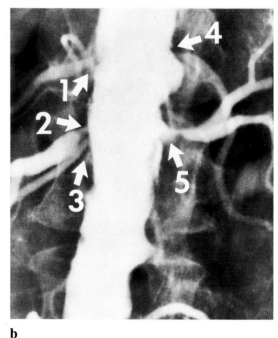

b

Fig. 8.13,a, b. Aortogram in two projections in a patient with severe hypertension and early kidney failure. **a** The customary P-A projection shows the two arteries to the left kidney (*4* and *5*) to be stenosed at their orifices. There are three arteries to the right kidney, but the orifices of the lower two (*2* and *3*) are obscured by the opacified aorta. Stenosis of the right upper pole branch is visible (*1*). **b** Aortogram with the patient rotated to her right shows orifice lesions in all three arteries to the right kidney (*1*, *2*, *3*). One can anticipate difficulty in performing a grafting operation to at least three and possibly four of the renal arteries. In the usual patient with this distribution of lesions, a transaortic endarterectomy is the ideal technique for rapid and simultaneous removal of all the obstructing

lesions. In this case, however, degenerative changes in the full length of the abdominal aortic wall can be anticipated and usually make endarterectomy confined to the pararenal aorta difficult to perform with safety. The urgency of the clinical situation mandated an aggressive approach. A supraceliac aortic clamp was used to avoid further disruption of the degenerated aortic intima and endarterectomy was successfully accomplished removing the aortic intima and the five orifice lesions as a single specimen. The aorta is still vulnerable to late aneurysm development and a preferable supplement to the operation would probably have been replacement of the infrarenal aorta with a prosthetic graft.

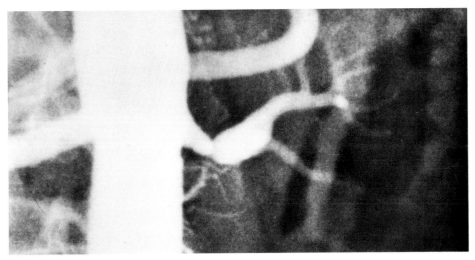

a

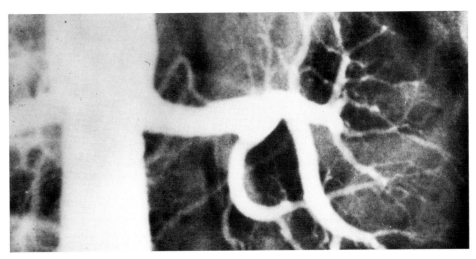

b

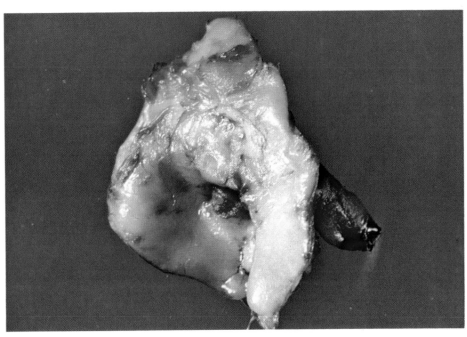

c

Fig. 8.14,a–c. Aortograms (**a** preoperative; **b** postoperative) and operative specimen (**c**) after trans-aortic unilateral renal endarterectomy. Inspection of the right renal orifice from within the aorta revealed a normal lumen at the orifice. A disc of thickened aortic intima twice the external diameter of the left renal artery has been removed in continuity with the renal artery lesions. This technique is also used for trans-subclavian endarterectomy of the right vertebral artery when disease is confined to the vertebral orifice.

247

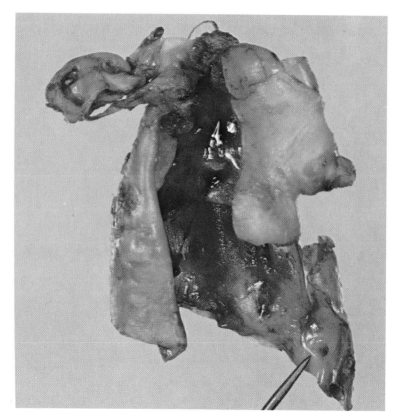

Fig. 8.15. Operative specimen removed by transaortic endarterectomy in a patient with atherosclerotic stenosis of both main renal arteries and an accessory left lower pole artery. The pointer indicates the stenotic orifice of the accessory artery.

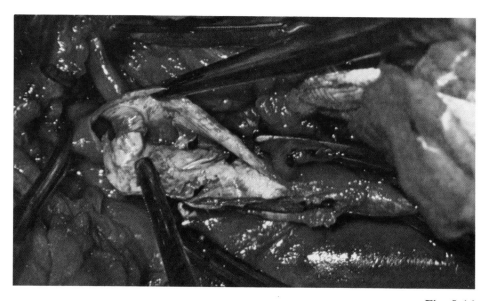

Fig. 8.16

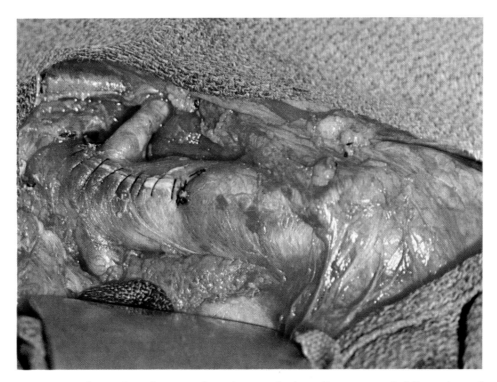

Fig. 8.17. Operative photograph at the conclusion of a transaortic bilateral renal endarterectomy (patient's head to the left). The color change in the renal arteries indicates the endarterectomy end points.

Fig. 8.16. Operative photograph of a transaortic renal endarterectomy in progress in a patient with bilateral renal artery stenosis due to atherosclerosis. Extensive infrarenal aortic stenosis was also present and was treated by aorta–common iliac endarterectomy. The renal portion of the operation was performed first. There was more than the usual distance between the SMA and the renal arteries, permitting the use of an infra-SMA position for the proximal occlusion of the aorta (clamp at the left). Also shown are the long aortotomy, the proximal level of transection of the aortic intima, and the prolapse of the right renal residual media into the aortic lumen as the intimal specimen is being withdrawn. Following the completion of a similar maneuver on the opposite side, the visible segment of the aortic intima is resected and the aortotomy closed to a level that permits relocation of the proximal aortic clamp to an infrarenal level.

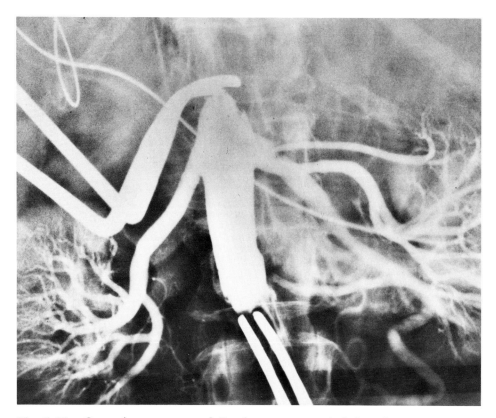

Fig. 8.18. Operative aortogram following a transaortic left endarterectomy. To obtain visualization of the renal arteries with adequate clarity and to avoid confusing the film with overlying shadows of the other visceral arteries and their branches, injection of contrast solution should be made into an isolated segment of the aorta.

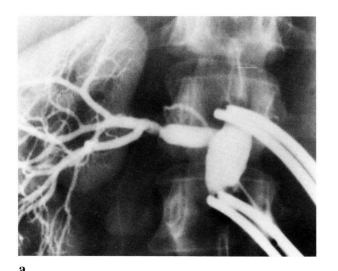

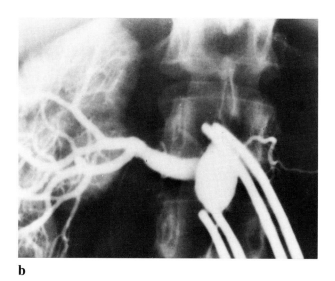

a   b

Fig. 8.19,a, b. Operative arteriograms following transaortic renal endarterectomy for atherosclerotic renal stenosis in a patient with a solitary right kidney. A distal intimal flap is shown in **a**; **b** shows the appearance of the artery after the flap has been removed through a distal transverse arteriotomy.

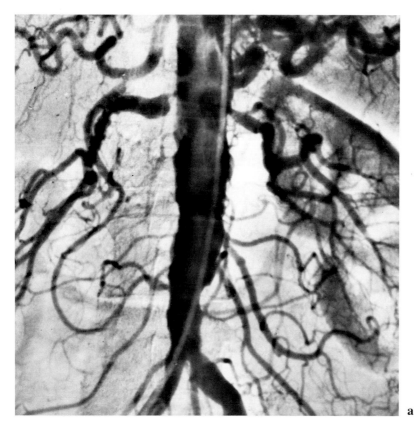

a

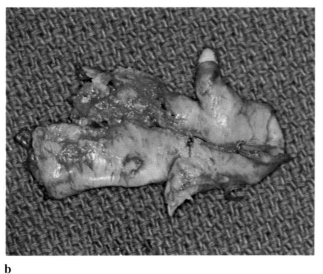

b

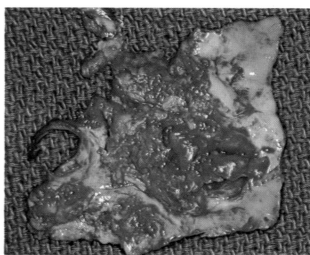

c

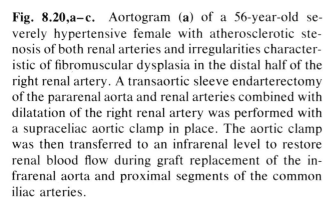

Fig. 8.20,a–c. Aortogram (**a**) of a 56-year-old severely hypertensive female with atherosclerotic stenosis of both renal arteries and irregularities characteristic of fibromuscular dysplasia in the distal half of the
right renal artery. A transaortic sleeve endarterectomy
of the pararenal aorta and renal arteries combined with
dilatation of the right renal artery was performed with
a supraceliac aortic clamp in place. The aortic clamp
was then transferred to an infrarenal level to restore
renal blood flow during graft replacement of the infrarenal aorta and proximal segments of the common
iliac arteries.

The irregular bulge of the aorta distal to the renal
arteries appearing at the customary level of the
beginning of an aortic aneurysm and the widening of
the common iliac arteries suggests medial degeneration and the probable accumulation of mural thrombus
and degenerating intima in the infrarenal aorta. An attempt at an anastomoses of grafts from such an aorta
to bypass the renal artery lesions is hazardous and ill-
advised.

In the endarterectomy specimen (**b** closed;
c opened), the endothelium surrounding the orifice of
the right renal artery (upper left corner of the opened
specimen) and the left renal artery (not visible) was intact, but ulceration and mural thrombus extends upward between the renal orifices.

An alternative operation that might have been
considered feasible from inspection of the aortogram
would have been graft replacement of the infrarenal
aorta, with an infrarenal clamp in place, followed by
the installation of bypass grafts from the sides of the
aortic prosthesis to the renal arteries. Inspection of the
specimen reveals the substantial risk of embolization
to the renal arteries that would have been incurred if
such an operation were to have been attempted.

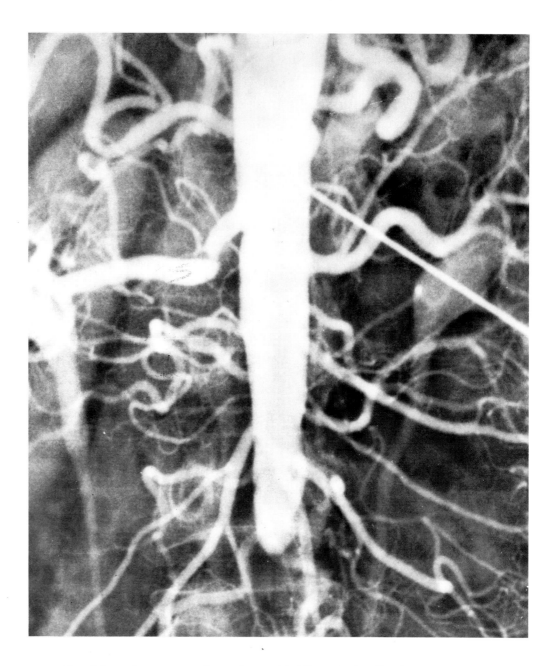

Fig. 8.21. Aortogram of a patient with bilateral claudication and hypertension. Atherosclerosis has occluded the aorta distal to the IMA. The tapered narrowing of the patent aortic segment is indicative of mural thrombus. A single right renal artery has an atherosclerotic stenosis 2 cm from its origin. A lower pole artery to the left kidney is stenosed at its origin from the aorta.

Transaortic endarterectomy of the right renal artery is feasible but difficult to perform because of the distal location of the renal lesion. The aorta (with its contained thrombus and the predictable atherosclerosis in its wall) is unsatisfactory for a proximal graft anastomosis to the right renal artery and the lower pole artery on the left side is too small to accept a distal anastomosis if a fabric graft were to be used.

Aortic endarterectomy with a suprarenal aortic clamp in place provided a smooth, thin-walled aorta to beyond the IMA and removed the stenotic lesion in the lower pole branch. The right renal artery was transected beyond the stenotic lesion and anastomosed to the side of the endarterectomized aorta. A bifurcation fabric graft was anastomosed to the aortic stump and its iliac arms extended to the common femoral arteries.

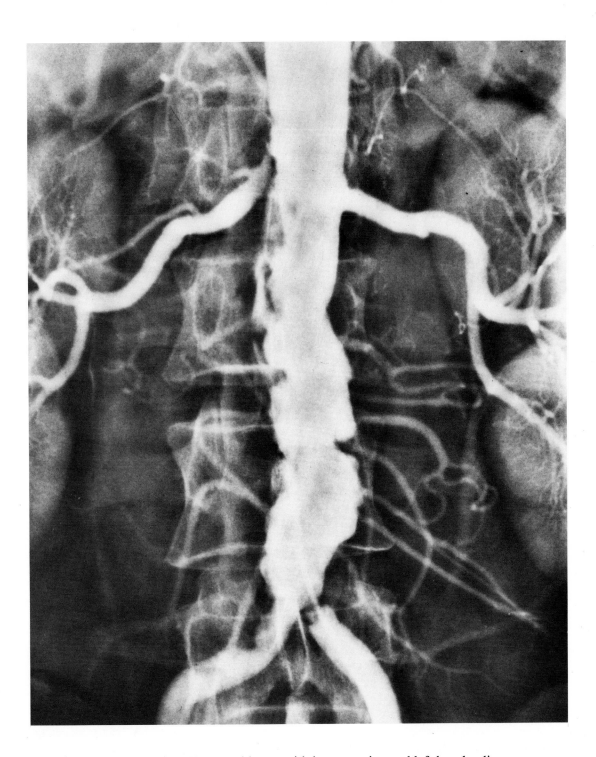

Fig. 8.22. Aortogram in a 53-year-old man with hypertension and left leg claudication showing stenosis of the right renal and the left common iliac arteries and
gross aneurysmal degenerative changes in the infrarenal aorta. The irregular contour of the right side of the aorta in the region of the origin of the right renal artery
suggests extensive intimal degeneration and mural thrombus. Endarterectomy is
feasible but difficult to perform, since the operation must also include graft replacement of the infrarenal aorta. The safest approach is an operation with supraceliac occlusion of the aorta in which the aorta is transected just below the origin
of the left renal artery. Easily detachable fragments are removed from the aortic
stump and a bifurcation graft is attached to it end-to-end. The right renal artery is
then transected at the appropriate level and anastomosed to the side of the graft.
The aneurysm is dealt with in the customary manner.

253

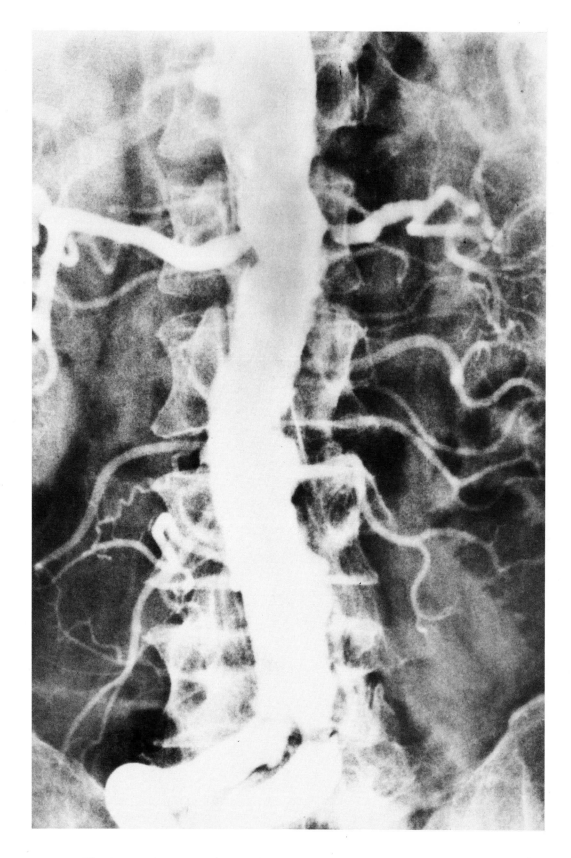

Fig. 8.23. Aortogram in a patient with renovascular hypertension, left renal artery stenosis, and diffuse degenerative preaneurysmal disease in the abdominal aorta. The probability of extensive granular intimal degeneration surrounding the renal orifices weighs against a satisfactory result from endarterectomy. The aorta was occluded at the supraceliac level. The infrarenal aorta was replaced by a bifurcation graft with a side arm to the left renal artery.

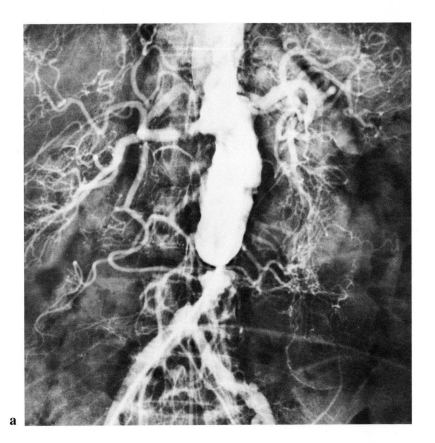

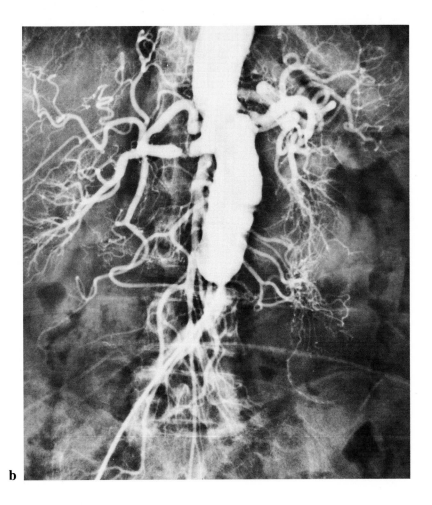

Fig. 8.24,a, b. Aortogram of a patient with atherosclerotic stenosis of the distal abdominal aorta and both renal arteries. Note the patulous contour of the infrarenal aorta. One can anticipate extensive intimal degeneration in the aorta, which precludes both transaortic renal endarterectomy and the use of the infrarenal aorta as the origin for a bypass graft. The operative technique therefore involved the use of a supraceliac aortic clamp and the preparation of an aortic bifurcation graft with 5-mm side-arm grafts sutured in position. The graft was anastomosed end-to-end to the aorta, which had been transected just distal to the SMA. The renal side arms were then anastomosed end-to-end to the transected middle thirds of the renal arteries.

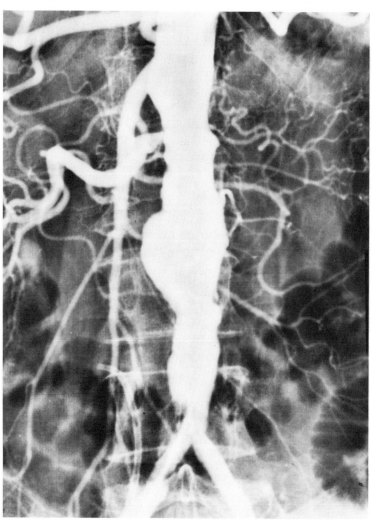

Fig. 8.25. Aortogram in a hypertensive patient with occlusion of the left renal artery, atherosclerotic stenosis of the right renal artery, and an aneurysm of the aorta. The mural thrombus that customarily lines the aneurysm has ascended to a level near the SMA orifice and surrounds the orifice of the right renal artery. The appropriate operation requires supraceliac clamping of the aorta, transection of the aorta below the SMA, anastomosis of a fabric graft to its proximal end, and reimplantation of the right renal artery into the side of the graft. The intimal degeneration associated with atherosclerotic aneurysmal disease precludes renal endarterectomy or even renal thrombectomy as reliable techniques for dealing with the stenotic lesion in the right renal artery.

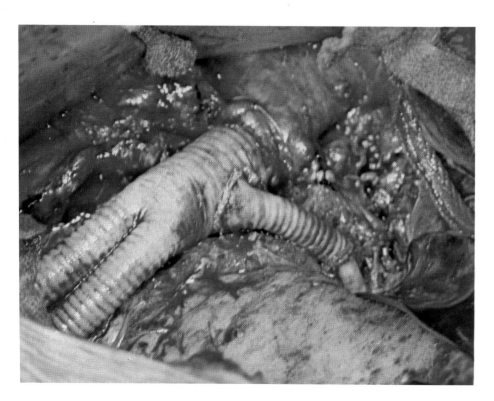

Fig. 8.26. Graft to left renal artery originating from an elliptical opening in the side of an aortic bifurcation graft. This was used in a patient with degenerative aneurysmal disease in the infrarenal aorta and atherosclerotic stenosis of the left renal artery. Note the bell-shaped beginning of the renal graft, which has been cut from a 12 × 6-mm bifurcation graft.

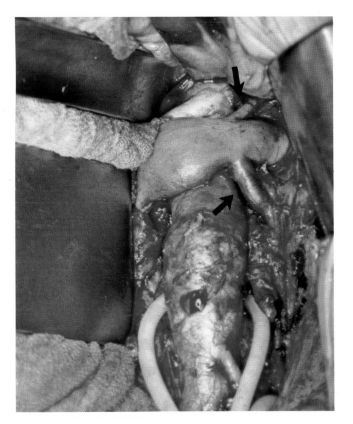

Fig. 8.27. Patulous aorta in a patient with hypertension secondary to bilateral atherosclerotic stenosis of the renal arteries. Perirenal granular degeneration of the aortic intima can be anticipated and becomes a contraindication to transaortic renal endarterectomy. Bypass grafts from the aorta to the renal arteries are contraindicated for the same reason and also because the bulge in the aorta may be the first stage in the development of a frank aneurysm.

At operation the aorta was clamped at the supraceliac level to avoid any possibility of renal embolization from a clamp on the aorta adjacent to the renal orifices. The aorta distal to the SMA was replaced with a tube graft to which side-arm grafts had previously been attached. These were then anastomosed end-to-end to the transected renal arteries.

In situations such as this, the exposure may be greatly enhanced by division of the left renal vein near its entrance into the vena cava. The left adrenal and the lumbar–gonadal veins (*arrows*) assist in retaining adequate venous drainage for the left kidney and should be preserved.

Index